OVER 40 &

Sexy a

THE COMPLETE GUIDE TO DIET, EXERCISE, SUPPLEMENTS, LIFESTYLE TRAINING, AND HOW YOUR BODY WORKS.

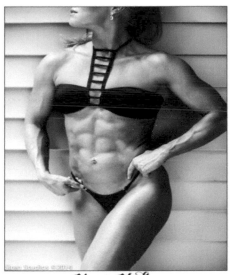

Siren Studios

ROBERT L. DRAPKIN, MD, FACP
with DONNY H. KIM, MASTER TRAINER, PES, CPT-NASM
and ASHLEIGH GASS, MS, CSCS, CCN, CNS, CISSN

Published by Richter Publishing LLC www.richterpublishing.com

Book Formatted By: Monica San Nicolas & Diana Fisler

ISBN:0692626727
ISBN-13:9780692626726

DISCLAIMER

This book is designed to provide information on health & fitness only. This information is provided and sold with the knowledge that the publisher and author do not offer any legal or medical advice. In the case of a need for any such expertise, consult with the appropriate professional. This book does not contain all information available on the subject. This book has not been created to be specific to any individual's or organization's situation or needs. Every effort has been made to make this book as accurate as possible. However, there may be typographical and/ or content errors. Therefore, this book should serve only as a general guide and not as the ultimate source of subject information. This book contains information that might be dated and is intended only to educate and entertain. The author and publisher shall have no liability or responsibility to any person or entity regarding any loss or damage incurred, or alleged to have incurred, directly or indirectly, by the information contained in this book. You hereby agree to be bound by this disclaimer or you may return this book within the guarantee time period for a full refund. In the interest of full disclosure, this book may contain affiliate links that might pay the authors a commission upon any purchase from the company. While the author and publisher take no responsibility for the business practices of these companies and or the performance of any product or service, the authors has used the product or service and makes a recommendation in good faith based on that experience. All characters appearing in this work are the authors themselves or clients who have given permission to use their story. Any resemblance any other real persons, living or dead, is purely coincidental. All photos and images have been provided by the authors by their resources & not that of the publisher.

CONTENTS

CHAPTER 1 The Most Important Thing.. 1

CHAPTER 2 Your Body Changes With Age 9

CHAPTER 3 How Your Body Works—Let's Start at the Beginning.......... 25

CHAPTER 4 DIET... 47

CHAPTER 5 EXERCISE 67

CHAPTER 6 How to Lose Fat and Build Muscle: Diet as it Relates to Exercise 112

CHAPTER 7 What is a Dietary Supplement? 118

CHAPTER 8 Over-the-Counter "Fat Burners"...................................... 134

CHAPTER 9 The Medical Management of Obesity From the Doctor's Point of View—Level II Data 136

CHAPTER 10 Evolution, Progress, Change 144

CHAPTER 11 Summary: How to Improve Your Health in 12 Steps 152

About the Authors 154

CHAPTER 1
THE MOST IMPORTANT THING

The most important thing in your life is your health. What were our reasons for writing this book? What's in this for you?

Why We Wrote This Book

I'm unhappy with the medical culture in the United States, because it focuses on treating the symptoms of the sick and does little to prevent the most common chronic diseases that are the leading causes of death and disability—and which are completely preventable! If you don't have the knowledge contained in this book, you'll likely develop a chronic metabolic illness and you'll be given prescription medications and likely told that it's part of "growing old" when, in fact, it is not.

The Centers for Disease Control and Prevention (CDC) clearly attest to this statement: lack of exercise, poor nutrition, tobacco use and alcohol cause much of the current chronic metabolic diseases, pain and early deaths. Most adults do not follow the CDC's recommendations.

Modern primary care physicians are trained to treat metabolic problems such as hypertension, adult-onset insulin resistant (type 2) diabetes, erectile dysfunction, coronary artery disease, stroke and dementia, yet few physicians provide detailed information on how to *prevent* these diseases—and this is truly the most important medical knowledge that everyone needs to have!

Society often does not like to rely upon human behavior to naturally correct social problems; this is why we have laws and police to enforce the laws. Maintaining good health through diet, exercise and up-to-date knowledge is ultimately the responsibility of each individual. What if this changed and the government decided that obesity was too expensive and cost too many lives, and they decided to intervene? This could happen insidiously—for example, too much sugar in some foods (this has been been attempted in New York City). What about, for example, a tax on obesity, along with higher healthcare insurance fees? Does this sound familiar?

The best solution is to read and follow the advice in this book, and become a good example of health through knowledge, to prevent and eliminate metabolic diseases.

Most patients today accept the minimal advice that their family doctors and nurse practitioners give them, and most patients take some of the pills prescribed to them. These medications—such as metformin, metoprolol and atorvastatin—are good medications, but they do not *cure* diseases. These pills palliate (lessen the severity of) diseases by hiding the signs of disease, giving patients a false sense of security and telling them that they can continue to live their unhealthy lifestyle. It's "OK" because "I take my blood pressure medication, my cholesterol medication and my pills for my elevated glucose."

The most difficult challenge today is *changing* your lifestyle and *eliminating the need* for these pills. The average American over 18 years of age fills 12 different prescriptions each year and takes over 10 pills per day. How many do you take?

The real benefit to removing hypertension, insulin-resistant diabetes and vascular diseases is that you'll live longer and feel stronger. Every organ in your body, including your brain, will perform better. Yes—even your sex life will improve.

I'm impressed with people who pay meticulous attention to their clothing. I'm impressed with the people who maintain their automobiles in spotless condition. I'm impressed with apartments and homes that have beautiful rooms and furniture. Why do we not pay meticulous attention to our bodies?

Mr. B's Story

Mr. B was born and raised in Chicago. He worked hard all his life and finally retired at age 65 and moved to Florida. When I first met Mr. B, his chief complaint was fatigue, loss his sex life, and weakness. His past medical history included high blood pressure, coronary artery disease with a stent placement, and poorly-controlled mature-onset (type 2) diabetes. His medications included metformin and insulin for his diabetes, a statin (even though his lipid profile was completely normal), two medications for his high blood pressure, and an anticoagulant. He saw his cardiologist and primary care physician on a regular basis.

On physical exam, his initial blood pressure was elevated at 169/98, and he weighed 226 pounds, with a BMI of 32, and was thus obese. His physical exam was otherwise normal, except for slight swelling in both lower extremities. Blood tests showed that his blood sugar was elevated at 160 mg/dl, despite his medications for diabetes, and he had mild kidney damage (creatinine 1.3/GFR 50ml/minute).

In summary, Mr. B had metabolic problems (see the section on metabolic syndrome). Furthermore, he had very low testosterone levels, and thus had testicular hypofunction.

Mr. B ate most of his meals at fast-food restaurants—his favorite was Taco Bell®. He snacked on candy bars, despite his diabetes. He had not done any exercising since high school. He did take all his medications, and felt secure that he was medically well, despite his dysfunctions. He asked me what I recommended.

I told Mr. B that he needed to lose body fat, and that this could best be done with a lower-calorie diet that was higher in protein, along with eliminating high-sugar-containing foods, averaging 1,600 calories— approximately 500 calories below his daily needs. I also found a personal trainer for Mr. B, and he started to exercise. I told him that if he could lose one pound per week and exercise three hours per week, then after four weeks I would consider prescribing supplements to return his hormone levels to normal.

After four weeks, Mr. B had made no progress whatsoever. He couldn't change his eating habits or lifestyle, and he quit the gym.

One year later, he came back to my office having suffered a heart attack (myocardial infarction). His problems had increased, despite the medications he'd been taking. He again asked me what to do, and I said, simply, "What you're doing now is not working! If you don't change, you'll continue to get worse."

We'll try again to help Mr. B and prevent further organ damage with diet and exercise to prolong his life. Interestingly, he drives a meticulously maintained eight-year-old car that looks "brand new," and lives in a perfectly maintained "model" home. His health is his most valuable possession, yet this is in poor condition.

Signs Your Body Needs Help

You have difficulty falling asleep. This is likely due to stress in your life and the subsequent elevation of the "stress hormone," cortisol. Sleep is your body's method of recovering from daily stress, but if the stress is too great, cortisol levels remain high and insomnia results. There are three possible solutions: one, to resolve the issues causing the stress; two, to relieve the stress through exercise, which lowers cortisol levels; or three, take a sleeping pill.

The stress-inducing issues may take a long time to resolve; exercise is therefore the best option, since it solves the problem quickly. Developing a pill habit leads to more potential complications.

You're getting shorter. Your height decreases because your bones are losing calcium due to a dietary lack of calcium (poor nutrition) or a Vitamin D deficiency. These nutritional deficiencies allow your spinal bones to flatten (compression fractures). Adult height loss can also be caused by curvature of the spine (kyphosis), which is due to nutritional deficiencies as noted above, as well as muscle weakness.

Your body is shaped like an apple, with your abdominal girth (waist size) bigger than your hip measurements. Visceral body fat is the fat that accumulates around your waist and correlates well with the development of metabolic diseases such as type 2 diabetes, hypertension and coronary heart disease. This problem can be solved only with both diet and exercise used together.

You have little energy. Fatigue can be caused by a variety of problems, such as low thyroid, low testosterone, poor nutrition, and/or abnormal metabolism. Your brain can decrease your metabolic rate. This problem can be handled with diet, exercise and the use of appropriate supplements.

My Story—What's in This for You?

The purpose of this book is to provide you with all the knowledge you'll need in order to improve your health and obtain the strength and vigor you once had, and to obtain the muscular body you once had (or wish to have). This text is a roadmap to good health and can take you beyond your expectations. I expect that since you're reading this, you're dissatisfied with your current body shape and you wish to do something about it. I was in your shoes at 48 years of age, and I had no idea how to change my life and become healthy.

What was happening to me in my forties has (or will) happen to you. I thought I knew how to eat healthy food and how to exercise. I thought I looked good. My wife and I went on vacation to Cozumel, Mexico. We rented a Jeep so we could go exploring and take photographs. In those days, we used film cameras and had to wait for the film to be developed before we could see the pictures.

On the next page is a picture of me during that vacation, at age 48.

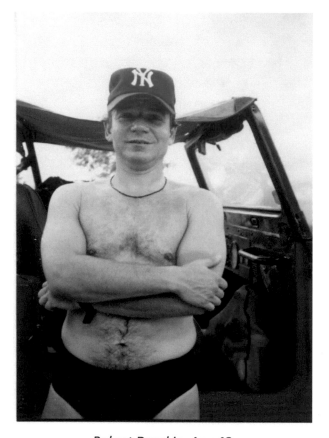

Robert Drapkin, Age 48

What's humorous about this is that I'd thought I looked good until the photo arrived, at which time I saw myself with a potbelly, a double chin, and a ridiculous attitude. This image was the stimulus for me to join a gym and restart my education, diet and exercise.

I joined a gym and attempted to "work out" on my own, as I was a physician and thought I knew "everything." In reality, I knew nothing, and for over two years, my body didn't change—my "love handles" stayed put, along with my double chin.

Then, by chance, I met Donny Kim, a certified personal trainer with a special interest in body mechanics and a champion bodybuilder. Donny started me on the road to good health, fitness and strength. We've remained good friends for 20 years, and now, with the help of Ashleigh Gass, we decided to put in writing all the knowledge we've learned on how to transform adults—both male and female—into strong, healthy and robust human beings.

If you decide to follow this roadmap, you'll feel the difference within three months, and see the difference within six months. Please take a photograph of yourself right now, get on the scale and weigh yourself, and measure your waist with a tape measure. Write down these numbers or store these data points on your mobile phone, and date the photograph. If you're unhappy with this photo and the numbers, you've just started on your road back to good health!

Below is an image of me at age 66—18 years later:

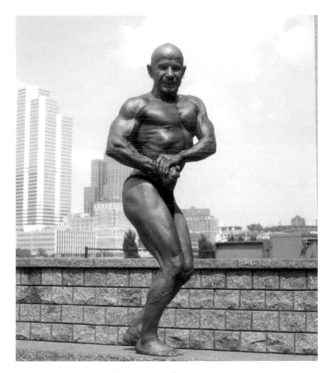

Robert Drapkin, Age 66

The Power to Change Behavior—Willpower

There are three essential components to long-term behavioral change. (Baumeister R, Tierney J (2011). *Willpower: Rediscovering the Greatest Human Strength*, New York, Penguin Press.)

1. You must have a goal;

2. You must be able to measure your progress; and

3. You must have willpower.

Willpower is the ability to postpone instant gratification in order to achieve a long-term goal. This involves the ability to control your impulses. Impulsivity involves an action that occurs with little or no planning or thinking, as opposed to actions that require careful thinking towards a planned outcome. The classic "marshmallow experiment" (Mischel W., et al. (2011). *Soc Cogn Affect Neurosci.* 6(2):252-256) showed that children able to delay gratification—one marshmallow now versus two marshmallows later—grew to be healthier and more successful adults. There are simple things you can do to increase your willpower:

1. Take slow, deep diaphragmatic breaths lasting 10 to 15 seconds per breath, which will decrease heart rate variability before you act. (Song HS, Lehrer PH (2003). *Appl Psychophys and Biofeed.* 28(1):13-23; Martarelli D, et al. (2011), *Evidence Based Compl and Alt Med.*)

2. Increase exercise. (Oaten M, Cheng K (2006). *Br J of H Psych.* 11:717-733.)

4. Work with successful people who have similar goals. (Fowler JH, Christakis NA (2008). *BML.* 87(1):337,2338.)

5. Wait for 10 minutes before taking action—change fast thinking to slow contemplation. (Bowen S, Marlatt A (2009). *Psych of Add Behavior.* 23(4):666-671.)

6. Think about your goals. (Noël X, et al. (2006). *How Your Brain Works—Decision-Making and Willpower. Psychiatry.* 3(5):30-41.)

CHAPTER 2
YOUR BODY CHANGES WITH AGE

We are born, we develop, we decline, and we die. The purpose of this book is to prolong the "develop" and delay the "decline" by understanding how your body works, and building muscle through exercise and diet. The most important aspect of good health and longevity is knowledge. The first part of this book will increase your understanding of how your body works. The second part of this book will outline the actions or path to building muscle, lowering body fat and increasing energy. In part three, you'll learn about supplements. Once you have this knowledge, you can create your own healthy lifestyle. We inherit the genes of our parents and we learn from our parents what to eat; we mimic their lifestyle (at least in early life). To improve, we need to learn from their mistakes and avail ourselves of more recently discovered information.

Today there is an epidemic of obesity leading to an epidemic of metabolic diseases. The National Institute of Health found that in 2009-2010, two out of three adults were overweight, with a BMI of 25-29.9; one out of three adults were obese, with a BMI 30-39.9; and one out of

20 adults were morbidly obese, with a BMI of 40+. (Flegal KM, et al. (2012). *JAMA*. 307(5):491-497.)

Morbid obesity is defined as a BMI greater than 40, and refers to a body that has medical problems due specifically to excess body fat. All of these problems can be prevented or lessened by using the knowledge presented in this book. Modern medicine prefers to palliate metabolic syndrome, hypertension, insulin resistant diabetes and hyperlipidemia with drugs. Yet, if you're motivated, learn from this book and understand your body, you'll enjoy a longer, healthier and more energetic life.

There are eight common changes in your body that occur between the ages of 40 to 60+, in addition to those changes associated with metabolic changes. These eight changes are familiar to all, and all can be treated or improved with diet, exercise and supplements: (1) memory loss; (2) bone and joint pain; (3) vision loss; (4) loss of skin elasticity; (5) frailty or muscular weakness due to muscle loss; (6) loss of sexual function/interest; (7) increase in body fat; and (8) loss of bone density.

(1) *Memory*. Exercise will help to improve your memory. (Erickson KI, et al. (2011). *PNAS*. 108(7):3017-3011.) In the elderly, the memory part of the brain—the hippocampus—shrinks in size as memory decreases. Exercise and nutrition increase the size of the hippocampus and cause memory improvement, thus reversing the effects of aging.

(2) *Bone and joint pain*. Obesity associated with aging is also significantly associated with increased osteoarthritis of the knees, due to the increased mechanical stress placed on the knees by increased body fat and the compensatory alterations in body mechanics. (Hartz A, et al. (1986). *J Chronic Diseases*. 39(4): 311-319.) By losing body fat, you can regain normal gait pattern ("gait" is the way you walk), and your knee pain will decrease. Strengthening core muscles is essential in eliminating lower back pain. Exercise and core muscle strength eliminate the need for back and knee surgery if started before serious damage occurs.

(3) *Vision loss*. Visual field loss is associated strongly with decreased mobility. (Turano KA, et al. (2004) *Optometry and Vision Science*.

81(5):298-307.) Another aspect of vision loss is small blood vessel damage associated with diabetes and insulin resistance caused by obesity and a sedentary lifestyle. If you prevent insulin resistance and prevent diabetes (as outlined in this book), you can save your vision.

(4) *Loss of skin elasticity*. We start losing muscle mass at age 30+, and we become weaker, more sedentary, and gain body fat. As growth hormones, androgen and estrogen levels diminish with age, we lose tissue elasticity, and wrinkles increase. (Makrantonaki E, Zouboulis CC (2007). *Experimental Gerontology*. 42(9):879-886.) Exercise and supplements are able to restore these hormone levels to normal values, thus reversing skin elasticity; wrinkles disappear and skin tightens back up. You won't need plastic surgery.

(5) *Frailty or muscular weakness due to muscle loss; (6) loss of sexual function/interest.* Loss of sexual interest and performance is a complicated issue involving multiple organ systems. Suffice it to say that exercise, diet and supplements will raise sex hormone levels to their normal ranges. If a hormone deficiency is the cause of the problem, this can be cured with knowledge, diet, exercise and supplements—doing what is written in this book.

If the problem is complicated by severe peripheral vascular disease, severe degenerative joint disease and/or myocardial muscle loss, it will be more difficult to correct.

(7) *Increase in body fat*. Body fat increases with age as you lose muscle mass starting in your thirties. You lose approximately 1% of muscle mass each year starting in your thirties, and by age 60, it's possible to have lost 30% of muscle tissue. This is discussed in detail later in this chapter.

(8) *Loss of bone density*. As you age, bone density decreases and you become shorter. Bone loss with age is common. Bone mass peaks at age 25 30 and then decreases slowly in both men and women. (O'Flarity HJ (1999). *Toxicology Sciences*. 55(1):171-188.) The amount of bone loss in the elderly is determined by many factors, including diet, exercise, calcium, Vitamin D, nutrition generally, hormone levels, gender, and genetics. Women have more rapid bone loss than men during their postmenopausal years, lasting five to 10 years. Postmenopausal women

also have a higher incidence of bone fracture than do men. Bone density is easily measured by a test called a dual-energy x ray absorptiometry (DEXA or DXA) bone density scan. This procedure is described in the next section of this book.

A DEXA scan will directly measure bone mineral density (BMD) and tell you a number (T score). If your T score is slightly below normal (1 to 2.5 standard deviations), you have osteopenia (mildly reduced bone mass), and need to take Vitamin D and calcium supplements, as well as increase your physical activity. If your T score is low (.2.5 standard deviations from normal), you have osteoporosis and you're at higher risk of bone fractures. You then need to take not only Vitamin D and calcium, but an additional medication-usually a bisphosphonate. Bisphosphonates prevent calcium loss in bones by blocking the cells (osteoclasts) that resorb bone. Exercise also prevents bone density loss. The purpose of these treatments is to prevent bone fractures.

John T's Story

John was a 50-year-old car salesman. He's been very successful in his career, but noticed that his younger competitors were becoming more successful. He had difficulty remembering customers' names. He noticed an increase in his waist size, and his shirts were tight around his neck. In the mornings, his knees hurt; e called this his "football knees." He began ending each day drinking scotch and smoking to better control the stress in his life. He lost interest in sex, due to his inability to perform. Even though he played varsity football in high school and understood the value of exercise, he hadn't exercised in 30 years. His diet consisted of fast food for breakfast and lunch, bar food for dinner. While driving home one evening, he was involved in a motor vehicle accident and injured his neck and lower back. His doctor told him that he had compression fractures in his spine and that he had osteopenia as shown by x-rays. This is when I first met John.

John had been admitted to the local hospital for trauma, anemia, a low platelet count, bone pain and an altered mental status. His blood pressure was elevated, he was obese, his blood sugar was high (consistent with adult onset diabetes), and he felt weak.

Within 48 hours, John had improved and wished to be discharged. He asked me one question: " How can I get my health back?" My answer was simple: "You've had an unhealthy lifestyle for 30 years. What you're doing is not working, and you're getting worse—not better. If you're willing to change your diet, exercise, stop smoking and decrease your alcohol intake, you'll get your health back."

John was lucky, because none of his metabolic problems were beyond repair. His high blood pressure and diabetes had not yet damaged his kidneys, and he hadn't had vascular injuries, such as heart attack or stroke, yet. He had degenerative joint disease, osteopenia and compression bone fractures—these did not require surgery. His anemia and low platelet count returned to normal levels with vitamin supplements and the discontinuation of alcohol.

With the proper knowledge, diet and exercise, all of his problems could return to normal—and they did. Within six months, he lost body fat, his waist size decreased by three inches, his blood pressure decreased, and his blood sugar returned to normal. His interest in the opposite sex returned when his free testosterone blood levels returned to normal. In addition, John's energy level increased, as did his car sales. Only his knees still hurt. John is now my life-long friend and patient.

What is Aging?

An aging cell loses the ability to divide and so dies. Cells are genetically programmed to divide a number of times. Cells collectively make up tissues and organs. These tissues and organs function only as well as their component cells. The testes, ovaries, kidneys and liver lose cell numbers relatively early in the aging body. The muscles, soft tissues and bones are among the first tissues to show measurable change.

It's difficult to define the "aging" process as distinct from disease or identifiable pathologic processes that can occur at any age. We do not know exactly what causes aging in every adult, but we've collected a significant amount of data to help explain some of the changes that occur as we age.

In general, distinct muscle changes usually occur in humans in the third decade. (Faulkner JA, et al. (2007). *Cl Exp Pharm Phys*. 34(11):1091-1096.) We lose 1% of our muscle mass on average every year starting at approximately age 30. Sedentary or inactive non-exercisers lose muscle mass more quickly. Data collected from healthy adults killed in automobile accidents shows significant age-related changes in skeletal muscle area and fiber content. We lose skeletal muscle mass as we age, and thus become weaker. Older muscle is also less efficient at protein synthesis than younger muscle of the same size and weight, and are thus weaker. This decrease in muscle mass and strength as we age leads to decreased activity. Decreased activity accelerates muscle loss.

This age-related change in muscle mass and strength alone leads to a less active lifestyle, continued muscle loss and a concomitant increase in body fat. (Waters DL, Baumgartner RN, Garry PJ (2000). *The Journal of Nutrition, Health & Aging*. 4(3):133-139.) It's a vicious, never-ending circle, and it will continue to worsen unless we interrupt the cycle with a change to a healthier life through diet, exercise and increased muscle mass.

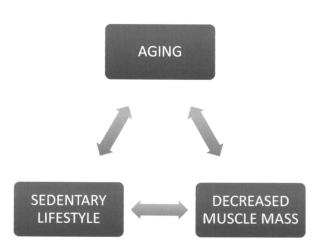

Body fat measurably increases as we age. The peak age for body fat mass occurs in adults aged 55 to 71 years. (Mott JW, et al. (1999). *Am J Clinical Nutrition*. 69(5):107-1013.) This is not inevitable, but it's totally up to you to do something about it.

Build Muscle at Any Age

It's possible to change this pattern of muscle loss with nutrition, exercise and normalizing hormones. Master athletes (defined as

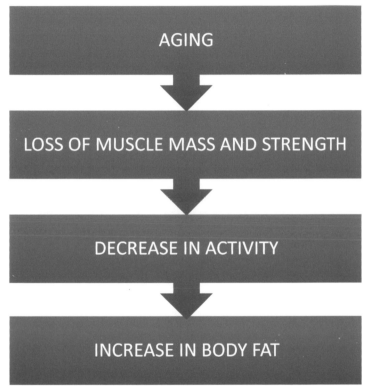

AGING

LOSS OF MUSCLE MASS AND STRENGTH

DECREASE IN ACTIVITY

INCREASE IN BODY FAT

performing vigorous exercises four to five times per week) aged 40 to 81 years had similar amounts of muscle mass and strength. (Wroblewski AP, et al. (2011). *Phys Sportsmed*. 39(3):172-178.) Thus, some of the decline in elderly muscle mass is due to chronic disuse—lack of exercise.

Nutrition is also very important, because protein is required for muscle development. In older muscle cells, higher levels of leucine and essential amino acids are required for muscle growth. (Fujita S, Volpi E (2006). *J Nutr*. 136(1):2775-2805.) Thus, a *high-protein diet* is *essential* for muscle growth.

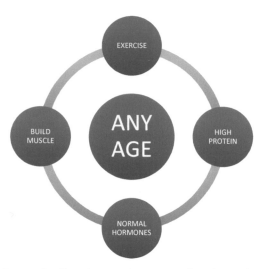

There is also a decline in sex hormone levels with aging. Men and women with low testosterone levels—regardless of cause—show a dramatic increase in muscle mass and loss of body fat when given testosterone supplements to return blood hormone levels to normal values. Vigorous exercise alone will increase both muscle mass and hormone levels. (Zemuda JM, et al. (1996). *Metabolism*. 45(8):935-939.)

Estrogen is also necessary for muscle growth. Estrogen stimulates "satellite cells" that repair damaged muscle cells, and stimulates new muscle growth. (Enns DL, Tildus PM (2008). *J Appl Physiol*. 104(2):347-353.)

Normal sex hormone and thyroid levels are necessary in both men and women for muscle growth. Optimal skeletal muscle growth occurs with testosterone levels in the upper levels of normal. It is my firm belief, based on the above studies and data, that it's possible to build muscle at any age with vigorous RESISTANCE TRAINING, SUPPLEMENTS, a HIGH-PROTEIN DIET, and NORMAL HORMONE LEVELS.

Unfortunately, there are no long-term studies of muscle growth in subjects over 30 years of age with stable sex hormone levels and vigorous exercise, leaving age as the only variable.

Even with the best training and advanced strength and mobility exercises to promote muscle growth at any age, your diet is important. A diet rich in plant and animal proteins and essential fats will ensure adequate amino acids essential for muscle growth, muscle recovery and optimal hormone levels. We'll discuss healthy carbohydrates in another section.

Additional and irrefutable evidence to support this concept are the photographs of bodybuilders in the master age groups of 40 to 80 years of age which are published online after each competition, available at http://musclepapa.smugmug.com.

Below is the body of a 70-year-old athlete:

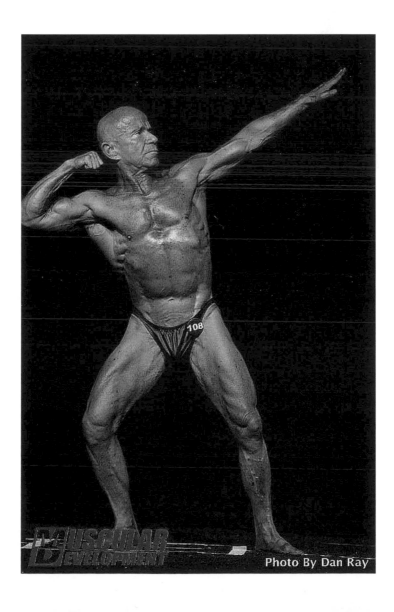

Photo By Dan Ray

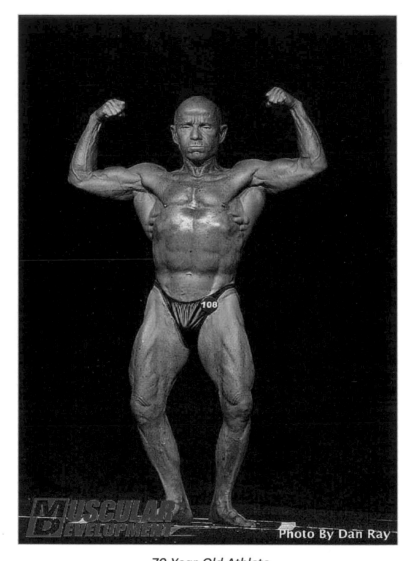

70-Year-Old Athlete

70-Year-Old Athlete
5.7% Body Fat After 500 Calorie Daily Reduction
for 90 Days—Caloric Restriction

Set a Higher Standard for Yourself

From my perspective as a professional trainer of both men and women, my first-hand experience tells me that anyone can get better at any age—*as long as you patiently maintain a healthy lifestyle with diet, exercise and supplements.*

This is truly the race won by the turtle. If you "let go" by smoking, excessive alcohol consumption and higher-caloric food intake, it's not simply the aging process that's making you fat—it's you. If you're in a hurry to lose weight and choose a "crash" ultra-low-calorie diet, you'll fail—you will lose fat and muscle and strength, and won't be able to *maintain* the fat loss. Your brain will automatically lower your metabolic rate. Your estrogen and testosterone levels will drop, and your cortisol (stress hormone) levels will increase, making you feel weak and depressed. (Cangemi R, et al. (2010). *Aging Cell.* 9(2):236-242; Tamiyama AJ et al. (2010). *Psychosomatic Medicine.* 72(4):357-364.) Your new behavior pattern is not sustainable, and you'll return to your previous bad habits.

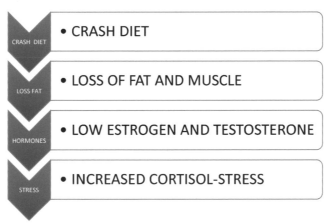

- CRASH DIET
- LOSS OF FAT AND MUSCLE
- LOW ESTROGEN AND TESTOSTERONE
- INCREASED CORTISOL-STRESS

In order to look younger, feel stronger and live longer, don't "let go." Think of yourself and your new lifestyle as a higher standard that sets you apart from your previous life.

Obesity Defined

Obesity has been defined as an abnormal accumulation of body fat—

approximately 20% or more of your ideal body weight. Ideal body weight is the weight for a specific age, gender and height that has the lowest death rate. This definition is more important for the life insurance industry than for you, because it doesn't take into account your body composition. How much of your body is bone, muscle or fat?

Body composition cannot be measured with a scale. Body composition is initially genetically determined. Obesity is also defined by a simple formula: body weight multiplied by 703 divided by twice the height in inches. This is your body mass index (BMI). A quick and simple way to determine your BMI is to use your iPad or other tablet and download "BOD keeper" app (bodkeeper.com). This app is very easy to use, and is essential, as you'll see later in this book.

A BMI of over 25 is considered overweight, and a BMI of 30 or more is obese. Again, this doesn't take body composition into account.

The Centers for Disease Control and Prevention calculates that 69% of adults over age 20 are overweight or obese.

Not every obese person has a metabolic problem, but most do, or will develop one. Asians have metabolic problems starting at a BMI of 25; Caucasians at 30; and African-Americans at 35. (Park YW, et al. (2003). *Arch Intern Med*. 163:427-436.)

In general, obesity is associated with an earlier death. (Fontaine KR, et al. (2003). *JAMA*. 289:187-193.)

Body fat is divided into two groups: subcutaneous fat (under the skin) and visceral body fat (around and inside organs, such as your liver). It's the visceral body fat that will shorten your life. (Huxley R, et al. (2010). *Eur J Clin Nutr*. 64:16-22.)

Subcutaneous body fat is often measured by skinfold calipers. You can purchase a skinfold caliper and measure skinfold thickness in several areas of your body. We prefer the seven-site procedure, which measures the following skinfold sites: abdomen; chest; mid-axilla; subscapularis; suprailiac; thigh; and triceps.

The numbers are added, and using formulas provided by the caliper manufacturer, your body fat can be calculated. The accuracy, if carefully done, will be within 4% of your true body fat.

This is a good measure to start with for most people, but in reality, you're not measuring visceral body fat. If you're athletic and have less

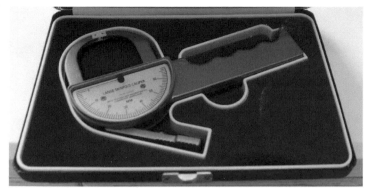

than 10% body fat, this method is not helpful. Visceral body fat loss can easily be measured by serial measurement of your waist size.

Lange Skinfold Calipers

The next best method of measuring total body fat is by using electrical impedance. A variety of devices are available (from inexpensive to expensive) that measure the resistance of body tissues to an electrical current. This measures total body water, and with this measurement and your weight, a calculation of body fat can be obtained. This technique is dependent upon body water, and your state of hydration will alter the results. This method is a good technique to start with, as long as your state of hydration is consistent.

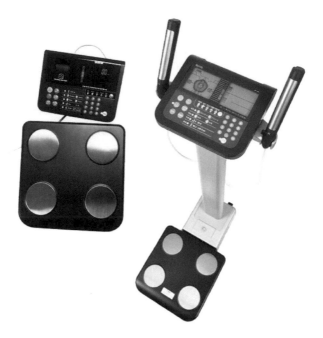

Tanita Electrical Impedance Devices

The most convenient and accurate method of measuring your body fat, muscle mass and bone density is with a DEXA (dual energy x ray absorptiometry) scan. This is a medical device that uses low-dose x rays to directly measure body composition. If you're athletic and are serious about body fat reduction, the DEXA scan is your best option.

I recommend a daily weight record and weekly waist size measurements to start, since these are the least expensive and are very reliable. If you can change your lifestyle for two weeks, these body measurements may give you more incentive to continue your journey to good health.

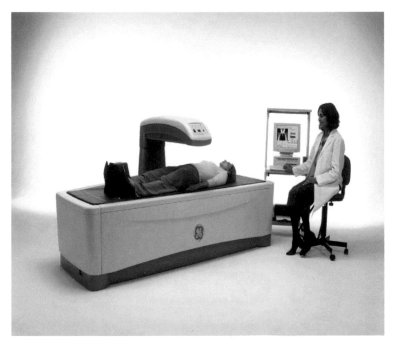

General Electric Dexa Scanner—Convenient and Accurate

Can Surgery Help Obese Patients?

Liposuction reduces subcutaneous fat, and the resulting loose skin can be surgically excised, resulting in a leaner-looking body. However, if an unhealthy lifestyle is the cause of the fat accumulation, surgery will not correct this behavioral problem, and the fat is likely to return over time unless the behavior is changed. Large volume liposuction does not alter a patient's risk for coronary artery disease. (Mohammed BS, et al. *Obesity*. 16, 120, 208:2648-2651.)

Bariatric surgery is currently a treatment for morbid obesity (BMI ≥ 40). Bariatric surgery can be restrictive; restrictive and malabsorptive; reversible; or permanent.

The most frequently performed procedure is a gastric bypass. This is a permanent operation that reduces the size of the stomach and connects this smaller stomach to a portion of the small bowel that bypasses two feet of normal small bowel. This is both restrictive and malabsorptive. Thus, the stomach holds less food, and the reduced size of the small intestine absorbs fewer nutrients.

The lap band procedure is a reversible procedure wherein an adjustable elastic band is placed around the upper portion of the stomach. This decreases the size of the stomach, and less food is able to be eaten.

Both procedures result in weight loss. Gastric bypass can improve insulin-resistant diabetes, but long-term studies show that these benefits will disappear in 24% of patients within three years. (DiGiorgi M, et al. (2010). *SOARD*. 6(3):249-253.)

Complications of gastric bypass include diarrhea, Vitamin B12 deficiency, iron deficiency, ulcers, secondary hyperparathyroidism, and pain. In one-year, three-year and five-year post-bariatric surgery follow-up, weight loss was found to be 76.8%, 69.7% and 56.1%; thus, weight gain occurs in a significant proportion of patients over time. (Golomb I, et al. (8/5/2015). *JAMA Surg.* 2202.)

It's difficult to treat a behavioral problem with surgery; an unhealthy lifestyle is the underlying problem, and this is not surgically correctable.

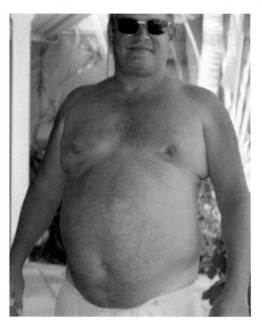

Visceral Body Fat—Is This You?

CHAPTER 3
HOW YOUR BODY WORKS—LET'S START AT THE BEGINNING

Diet—What You Eat

The most important part of your healthy diet is your knowledge of food and of how your body uses food to create body fat and muscle and prevent disease. Most of us learn about food from our parents, and we all assume that we know what's healthy to eat. Because most people have no idea of which foods are healthy, insulin-resistant diabetes, heart disease and obesity are major health problems. Do fat parents have fat children? The answer to this is unequivocally "yes." (Manios Y, et al. (2007). *BioMed Central Public Health*. 7:178.) Do most parents recognize this? No. What is missing is knowledge.

There is no diet that fits all people equally. Your food choices are part of a healthy lifestyle that achieves your goals and continues over your entire life. Your diet is a pathway to a lifetime of health. Your diet should not be a race to lose weight—but if it *were* a race, it's a race won by the turtle and not the hare. Think of your diet as one small daily step towards your goals.

Digestion

Food can be classified as proteins, carbohydrates, fats, fiber and micronutrients (vitamins and minerals). You put food in your mouth. You chew your food into smaller bits and swallow, and the mix enters your stomach.

Once in the stomach, hydrochloric acid (HCl) continues the process of breaking the food into smaller bits. HCl is very important, because it breaks down proteins into amino acids, activates other digestive enzymes, and prevents bacterial overgrowth. Both stomach HCl production and digestive enzyme production decrease after age 65. (Feldman M, et al. (1996). *Gastroenterology*. 110, 40:1043-1052.) This decrease may cause indigestion and heartburn; thus, not all stomach problems are caused by *increased* stomach acid, and antacid medication is *not* universally helpful.

The mix of food then enters the small intestine, where the digestive process is completed. Enzymes digest proteins into amino acids, fats into fatty acids, and carbohydrates into simple sugars (glucose and fructose). Fiber in the mix slows the rate of absorption of some of these nutrients; fiber itself is not digested.

The mix of amino acids, sugars and fatty acids then goes directly to the liver via the hepatic portal vein for immediate use, and also enters the bloodstream. The pancreas detects these three classes of nutrients (macronutrients) in the blood, and releases insulin to remove these nutrients. Insulin converts sugars into fat and liver glycogen; amino acids are assembled into muscle; and fat is converted to fatty acids which are stored in fat cells as triglycerides.

What is a Calorie?

A calorie is a unit of measure that has been applied to all food groups. A calorie has been defined as the amount of heat required to raise one kg of water by one degree centigrade. Thus, the relative energy value of all foods can be measured in a science lab. Your body, however, does not metabolize all food groups in the same manner, and calorie content is not the best measure of food value. It's more important to know how your body uses each type of food macronutrient (fat, protein and carbohydrates). Calories are useful to find a starting point for your diet and a general plan for each type of

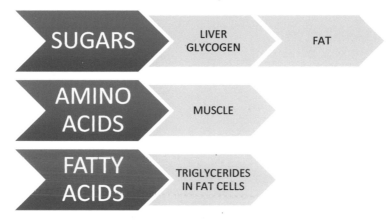

food, but the bottom line in a healthy diet is that to lose body fat, you must consume fewer calories than your body burns.

Fat in the Diet is Essential

Fat in the diet is essential. You must have fat in your diet.

Fat is a source of energy for cells, containing 9 calories per gram as compared to the 4 calories per gram that both carbohydrates and protein contain. Yet it is not the fat in your diet that makes most of your body fat.

Fat is a component of every cell membrane and is thus necessary for healthy tissues. It's a component of nerve cells, and is essential for nerve conduction and brain function. All steroid hormone synthesis (testosterone and estrogens) is based on the cholesterol molecule, and cholesterol is an essential fat. The most recent data suggests there is no link between saturated fat consumption and heart disease, diabetes or obesity. (Teicholz N. *The Big Fat Surprise*, Simon and Schuster, 2014.)

There is one group of dietary fats that are unhealthy without controversy—trans fats. Trans fats are usually man-made saturated fats produced by hydrogenating vegetable oils. These trans fats do not spoil quickly and so produce products that have longer commercial shelf lives. Trans fats have been used to make margarine and packaged baked goods such as cookies, crackers and snack cakes. All man-made trans fats have been proven to increase the risk of cardiovascular disease, and the U.S. Food and Drug Administration (FDA) is in the process of eliminating trans fats from the food supply. Always check product labels on your packaged foods for trans fats.

Body Fat and Sugar—How You Become Fat

The more sugar in the blood, the higher the insulin levels and, thus, the greater production of fat. When insulin levels are low, triglycerides

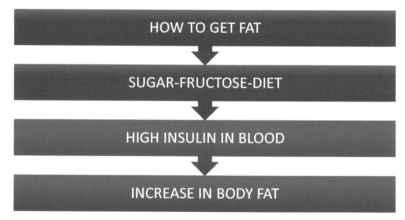

residing inside fat cells get broken down into fatty acids for energy, and the fat cells shrink in size—this is a decrease in body fat.

Hormones control the speed that these metabolic processes occur— from the hypothalamic portion of the brain, from the pituitary gland, and from the thyroid gland.

Leptin, a hormone produced by fat cells, helps the body regulate energy balance by inhibiting the sensation of hunger. When leptin is released into the bloodstream, it tells the brain that you have enough

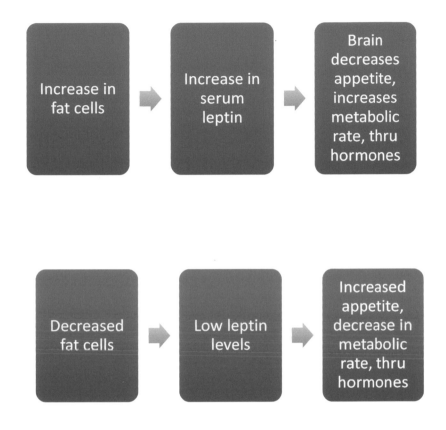

energy stored as fat and to reduce appetite. Low leptin levels tell the brain that food intake is low and so the brain slows down the body's rate of energy consumption (metabolic rate). The body tries to maintain a steady state (homeostasis), and when fat is high, leptin is high, and the metabolic rate increases to compensate for the increased energy available. When fat is low, leptin decreases and again attempts to keep the body constant by decreasing the metabolic rate.

Serum leptin levels correlate with body fat levels, and can be used as a measure of your body fat.

How Your Body Works

Your body muscles and organs require a source of energy while the fat cells store and save energy. High insulin levels direct macronutrients into storage, while low insulin levels direct nutrients into direct use for energy. A new finding reveals that high insulin levels can block leptin function and cause both a low metabolic rate and simultaneous fat storage. The presence of high insulin levels is the real problem, since insulin creates body fat. With high insulin levels, the leptin signal causes no decrease in appetite, and energy expenditures do not increase. This is how we become obese and morbidly obese.

It is possible to change this. Here are a few simple steps to take:

1. Decrease insulin production by eliminating foods with high sugar content and low fiber content, such as juice, cakes, pies, candy, milk products, soft drinks, bread and pasta.

2. Consume protein foods with each meal to increase satiety.

3. Increase intake of foods with fiber, such as all vegetables and salads, to slow the absorption of all nutrients.

4. Increase exercise and increase the number and quality of the mitochondria inside your muscle cells, building more muscle cells and thus increasing your metabolic rate. More muscles = more calories burned while you rest.

5. Stress reduction and adequate sleep will lower insulin levels by decreasing cortisol production—refer to the section on cortisol and stress.

In summary, high insulin levels determine whether we become fat, by blocking leptin and by creating body fat. The number and size of fat cells determine your body fat. You make fat cells during the first two years of life, and this is determined by factors beyond your control. However, the *contents* of these fat cells is under your control, and is determined by insulin; the more insulin you make, the more fat is stored in your fat cells.

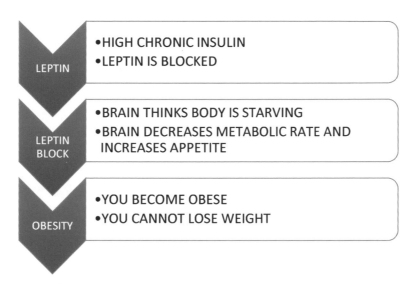

It is very important to decrease insulin levels and to decrease your total body fat by way of a diet low in sugars and a lifestyle that burns sugars and builds muscle through exercise. Sugar calories are, thus, the dangerous calories.

We need some fat as a healthy source of energy, but modern lifestyles and certain foods lead to disease. Let's return to the digested food in the small intestine. Carbohydrates are broken down into glucose and then released into the bloodstream.

The liver now converts some of this glucose into glycogen (a healthy form of energy storage in the liver). Fat in the small intestine is converted into fatty acids. Fatty acids are processed by the liver and linked to lipoproteins so that they can be transported to all the cells in the body and then used as an energy source or be stored in fat cells.

Protein in the diet is converted into amino acids in the small intestine and is used to build and maintain muscle cells. Any excess is converted into fat by the liver, as well, but this process consumes as much energy as it produces. Thus, the liver must deal with the excesses in our diet.

When glycogen storage in the liver is full, this fat must be stored outside the liver in fat cells, the majority of which are located in your abdomen as visceral body fat. Some of this fat is also stored under your skin as subcutaneous body fat. Thus, excessive caloric intake *does* count and *does* lead to body fat.

Stress and Bad Behavior

Stress is a physiological and biochemical event that occurs when your brain perceives a threat. Stress ultimately causes the release of cortisol by the adrenal glands. Other hormones may be released, as well, including norepinephrine, epinephrine, testosterone and estrogen. Stress begins in the brain and affects the entire body. The elevated cortisol levels cause an increase in appetite by increasing activity in the parasympathetic nervous system and the vagus nerve. Cortisol increases blood pressure and blood glucose.

We all experience stress, and some people experience more stress than others. When stress is transient, the cortisol level returns to normal, and all is well. Prolonged stress is harmful. It is chronic or prolonged stress that really creates problems. Prolonged elevated cortisol levels raise blood glucose and, subsequently, insulin levels. Eventually, the body's cells stop responding to the constantly elevated insulin (this is known as "insulin resistance"). Insulin resistance causes a variety of metabolic problems that we will discuss later.

Stress also causes insomnia, and the brain interprets this as an additional stress and so causes even more cortisol to be produced. With chronic cortisol overproduction, blood sugar increases, as do insulin levels. The insulin blocks the effect of leptin on the brain, and the brain sees only low leptin levels and so increases appetite. (Mietus-Snyder ML, et al. (2008). *Ann Rev Med.* 59:119-134.)

Again, a high insulin level produces fat, and low leptin function decreases the metabolic rate, and so we get fatter.

	• STRESSFUL SITUATION
STRESS	• CORTISOL RELEASED BY ADRENAL GLANDS

	• INCREASED APPETITE
INCREASED APPETITE	• INCREASED BLOOD SUGAR

	• INCREASED INSULIN
INSULIN	• BODY MAKES FAT

Big Mike's Story

Big Mike is a patient of mine with chronic high insulin levels. Mike is morbidly obese, with a large, protruding belly (high visceral body fat). Early in life, he developed very bad eating habits. Eating food became his way of reducing stress. Whenever life became difficult, Mike would eat something sweet to provide immediate stress relief and pleasure. This pattern of behavior became his pattern of life. This fixation with food was a severe psychological problem, with inevitable results. He would chronically over eat, drinking a gallon of whole milk every day and enjoying high-calorie desserts every day. He enjoyed a sedentary lifestyle, and at an early age, he developed insulin resistant-diabetes.

His pancreas stopped producing high insulin levels and his blood sugar became constantly elevated. Instead of changing his diet, he was placed on insulin injections by his family doctor. This did return his blood sugar to a more normal level, and so allowed Mike to continue overeating.

Eventually, his belly became so large that he had to change the position of his back and hips in order to walk upright. This alteration in his gait led to severe lower back and neck pain, as well as severe degenerative joint disease. Today, Mike is unable to walk. He continues to overeat and self-medicate with insulin. He is essentially homebound, despite being under 70 years of age.

If you find yourself using food for emotional stress relief on a regular basis, here are some suggestions:

1. Don't purchase or possess any of the foods that you usually use for stress reduction or pleasure.

2. Plan and prepare all your meals in advance, and eat each meal at a defined or specific time.

3. Find a different activity for stress relief. The best and most effective stress-relieving activity is exercise. Other stress-relieving activities include computer use, reading books, massage, shopping, meditation, yoga and Pilates. None of these activities will make you obese.

Why Body Fat is Bad

As your body ages, it's the excess body fat that increases the risk of hypertension, insulin-resistant diabetes, coronary artery disease, stroke, dementia, and bone and joint injury. (Guo SS, et al. (2007). *Am J Physiol.* 1041-1051; Guo SS, et al. (1999). *Am J Clin Nutr.* 70:405-411.)

Fatty tissue makes up a large percentage of the cells in your body. Men average between 18-24% body fat; women average between 25-31% body fat. Fat cells can become "dysfunctional" and accelerate age-related diseases, while one's life span is extended by caloric restriction and a reduction in visceral fat. (Ahima RS (2009). *Connecting obesity, aging and diabetes. Nat Med.* 15:996-997.) Fat cells store energy—fatty acids in the form of triglycerides. Fatty tissue is located beneath the skin (subcutaneous) and around vital organs (visceral). Fatty tissue produces hormones and cytokines that affect body temperature, immune function, wound healing and sex. It is theorized that with increased fat cell replication, fat cell precursors become dysfunctional with age, and in the presence of chronic high insulin levels produce inflammatory products (tumor necrosis factors) that damage blood vessels and other tissues, causing the pathologies associated with obesity and age. (Tchkonia et al. (2010). *Aging Cell.* 9:667-684; Xu et al. (12/15/2003). *J Clin Invest.* 112(12):1821-1830.)

Statistics from the NIH reveal a 14 year reduction in life expectancy in extremely obese adults. The reason that fat people die younger can be attributed to insulin resistance in the cells of the liver and the development of metabolic syndromes.

Ligands, Insulin Resistance and Metabolic Syndromes

All biologic systems depend upon the ability of cells to communicate. Cells communicate by using messages called ligands. Ligands are molecules that bind to other molecules to create a new effect. Ligands released into the circulation seek out specific cells by looking for specific "receptors" on cell surfaces. The desired communication between cells occurs when a cell surface membrane receptor and a chemical ligand come together. The result of the binding of a ligand to a cell receptor is a new activity or new protein in the cell.

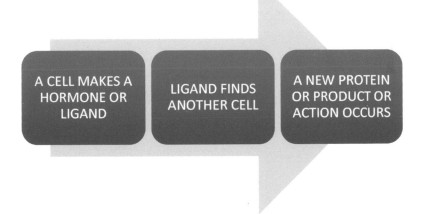

This is how your cells communicate:

The cell receptors are metabolically active and can increase in number as more ligands are presented. It is also possible that in the presence of excess ligands, the receptor activity can decrease or become resistant. The precise reason that human cells become resistant to excess insulin is not known, but the results of this *are* known: insulin resistance results in higher blood sugar levels. The pancreas detects this increase in sugar and produces more insulin, making things even worse. Eventually, the cells of the pancreas fail because they are overworked, and diabetes results.

The liver decreases the storage of sugar by decreasing the production of glycogen from glucose. Insulin-resistant fat cells no longer take up circulating lipids, and increase the fatty acids in circulation, leading to elevated serum triglycerides. Fat cells lose the ability to store triglycerides. These abnormal lipids in the bloodstream—specifically small, dense, low-density lipoproteins (LDL)—stick to and damage the walls of arteries, thus producing arterial disease throughout the body.

Insulin resistance is associated with the presence of increased blood pressure (hypertension). Approximately 50% of people with hypertension are insulin-resistant. (*J Clin Invest*. (2000) 106(4):453-458.)

In non-insulin-resistant people, insulin causes dilatation of blood vessels. In insulin-resistant people, no dilatation occurs, due to the failure of cells in the blood vessel linings to release nitric oxide. The smooth muscle cells surrounding the blood vessels restrict blood flow, causing a compensatory increase in pressure. Blood flow is ultimately decreased. (Laakso M et al. (1990). *J Clin Invest*. 85:1844-1852.) This is also how we develop hypertension, erectile dysfunction in men, peripheral vascular disease and coronary artery disease. Poor blood flow to the penis or vagina affects a person's ability to become aroused and have sexual intercourse.

Nitric oxide in pill form can be increased to palliate these conditions, such as in nitroglycerin pills, sildenafil (Viagra, etc.), and a variety of over-the-counter supplements.

Metabolic Syndromes and Organ Damage Caused by Chronic Insulin Overproduction

1. High blood pressure (hypertension);

2. High blood sugar (type 2 or adult onset diabetes);

3. Abnormal lipids (hyperlipidemia)—elevated LDL;

4.   Coronary artery disease (heart disease);

5.   Peripheral vascular disease;

6.   Stroke (brain damage);

7.   Kidney damage.

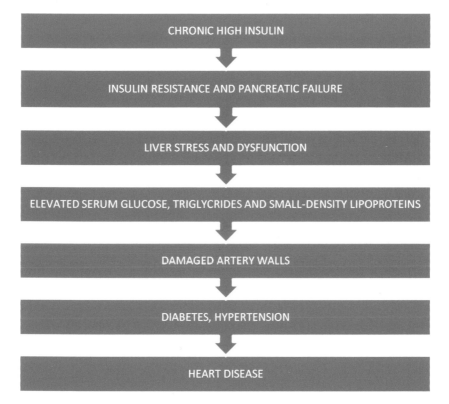

The "metabolic syndrome" is a group of medical conditions defined by the presence of any three of these conditions: high blood sugar; high triglycerides; low high-density lipoproteins (HDL); visceral obesity; and hypertension. Approximately 34% of Americans have metabolic syndrome. (Ford ES, et al. (2002). *JAMA*. 287(3):356-359.)

Metabolic syndrome is a precursor leading to diabetes, heart disease and death. You don't die from obesity, but you will eventually die from its resultant metabolic syndromes.

Carbohydrates are Essential and Complicated

Carbohydrates are the sugars that are the main source of energy for your cells. Plants produce carbohydrates. The sugar in your blood is glucose. Your food contains many different forms of carbohydrates: fructose is the sugar in fruit; galactose is the sugar in milk; table sugar or sucrose contains one unit of glucose and one unit of fructose; starch contains many units of glucose (polysaccharide); fiber is comprised of carbohydrates that are not digested.

Carbohydrates are digested in the stomach and small intestine into sugars (glucose and fructose). When glucose enters the bloodstream, insulin is secreted by the pancreas, and glucose then enters all of the body's living cells, where it's immediately used as an energy source. Glucose can be stored in the liver as glycogen for future use. Excess glucose not burned for energy, nor stored as glycogen in the liver or muscles, is converted to triglycerides and stored in fat cells.

The liver can store between 80-100 grams of glycogen, and the muscles in the body can store 300-600 grams of glycogen (depending on total body muscle mass).

Fructose occurs in fruit and is always combined with glucose. Fructose is more harmful than glucose, because fructose can only be metabolized by liver cells and not by any other body cells. Fructose in excess is not converted to benign glycogen, but is converted to fatty acids, triglycerides, and harmful low-density lipoproteins. (Mayes PA (1993). *Am J Clin Nut*. 58(5):7545-7655.) This leads to insulin resistance, and thus, your 12 ounce glass of orange juice in the morning is just as unhealthy as 12 ounces of Coca-Cola. (Actually, the drink has less fructose, and may prove to be healthier.) Alcohol (ethanol) is even worse, since it can cause direct cell damage to the brain and heart, in addition to requiring liver-only metabolism such as does fructose.

The ability of a carbohydrate to enter the bloodstream as glucose can be measured relative to pure glucose, and this is called the "glycemic index." A high-glycemic index food, such as white bread, elevates your blood glucose level faster and much higher than does a low-glycemic carbohydrate, such as broccoli. Fiber is an important aspect of glycemic index, since high fiber reduces the glycemic load of foods by delaying absorption of food in the small intestine.

Fiber is a plant product (carbohydrate) that humans cannot digest. It is beneficial in slowing the absorption rate of nutrients (sugars and fats). This slower rate of glucose absorption lowers peak insulin levels and helps to maintain lower insulin levels. The slower the absorption of fructose, the lower the amount of metabolic stress on the liver. The delayed fat absorption moves fat into the colon, where it can be eliminated. Sugars are used by cells for energy or are stored as fat, but they are never eliminated. You either burn sugar or you wear it.

The fiber in fruit allows the fruit to be a healthier food, because the sugar (fructose) is more slowly absorbed, and peak insulin levels are therefore lower. Eat the fruit but don't drink the juice—juice contains lots of sugar but no fiber.

An additional source of fiber frequently overlooked is flax meal. Flax meal is made from finely-ground flax seeds and provides fiber and omega 3 fatty acids. We recommend two tablespoons of flax meal daily.

Protein

Protein is present in the inner and outer portion of every cell. Cells make up your tissues. Your body can store fats and carbohydrates, but not protein. The protein in your food (poultry, fish, beef, dairy, and some plants) is broken down into amino acids in the stomach and small intestine. These amino acids are then reassembled into the tissues of your body relatively quickly. Your body is in constant repair and renewal of tissues, and needs amino acids to do this work.

According to Dr. Jonas Frisen, your body (with the exception of the brain) renews itself completely every seven to 10 years. The liver converts excess amino acids into glucose or fat. Exercise causes muscle growth and muscle repair, and increases the need for protein in the diet. Exercise in the absence of sufficient amino acids can cause tissue damage. If you exercise, you need to eat enough protein to maintain or improve your muscles.

C-Reactive Protein

C-reactive protein (CRP) is made by the liver in response to ligands or products produced by white blood cells (macrophages) and fat cells. This is usually in the presence of dying or injured cells, and CRP activates the innate immune system (a complementary system) found in the liver to help the body remove dead cells. CRP elevations can occur with exposure to environmental toxins and diets rich in heavy metals and trans fat.

CRP decreases with any long-term increase in exercise. Exercise reduces the incidence of coronary artery disease, and this decrease in CRP may be part of the reason exercise is beneficial. (Kasapis C, Thompson PD (2005). *JACC*. 45(10):1563-1569.)

Dietary Fat

Approximately 20-30% of your dietary calories should come from the fat in your diet. Dietary fat is an important source of fuel for the cells of the body, providing 9 calories per gram of fat, while carbohydrates and proteins provide only 4 calories per gram. Fats are a very important part of your diet.

The fat-soluble vitamins (A, D, E and K) are essential dietary nutrients found in the liver and fatty tissues of animals. Fats (glycerophospholipids) are the main structural component of all biologic cell membranes. All steroid hormones, including cortisol, estrogen and testosterone, are made from lipids.

All of the fat in your food is comprised of combinations of fatty acids that differ in the number of hydrogen atoms attached to the carbon atoms. A saturated fat, such as butter, has more hydrogen atoms than does a monounsaturated fat, such as olive oil. Unsaturated fats are found in plants, vegetable oils, seeds, fish and nuts. Saturated fats are the fats found in animal meat, dairy products, coconut products and palm products.

The digestion of fat in the small intestine is complex and requires the presence of lipase, bile salts, phospholipids and transport lipoproteins.

The dietary fat is broken down into triglycerides and fatty acids. Fatty acids can be stored in fat cells and can be used as a source of energy. Once inside the cells of the small intestine, the fatty acids, cholesterol, and fat-soluble vitamins form chylomicrons that allow fat to enter the lymphatic circulation and subsequently the large veins of the chest, and then into the liver. (Chylomicrons are lipoprotein particles consisting of triglycerides (85 92%), phospholipids (6 12%), cholesterol (1 3%) and proteins (1 2%); they transport dietary lipids from the intestines to other locations in the body.)

Unsaturated Fats

OLIVE, NUT AND CANOLA OILS

NUTS: ALMONDS, WALNUTS, PECANS

AVOCADOS AND SEEDS

FISH

Saturated Fats

ANIMAL MEAT: BEEF, CHICKEN, PORK

MILK PRODUCTS, CHEESE

COCONUT AND PALM PRODUCTS

Fat—Measured by Blood Tests

Fat is not water-soluble and cannot circulate in the bloodstream unless it's converted into a lipoprotein complex by the liver. These lipoprotein complexes are measured by blood tests called lipid profiles.

Fats processed and released as "carriers of lipids," called "apolipoproteins," are classified according to their density: very low-density lipoproteins (VLDL) carry newly-synthesized triglycerides from the liver to fat cells for energy storage; low-density lipoproteins (LDL) carry phospholipids, cholesterol and triglycerides throughout the body to cells for repair and for energy; high-density lipoproteins (HDL) transport phospholipids, cholesterol and triglycerides from the cells of the body back to the liver.

The size of LDL particles varies from large and buoyant to small and dense. Small, dense LDL is especially rich in cholesterol and is associated with atherosclerotic heart disease and other diseases of vascular damage. The increased pathology of small, dense LDL derives from less-efficient hepatic LDL receptor binding, leading to prolonged circulation and exposure to endothelium and increased oxidation.

Apolipoprotein synthesis in the liver is controlled by many factors: dietary composition, alcohol, fructose, hormones, vitamins and drugs. When stressed by dietary excesses, such as alcohol, trans fats, high insulin levels, and medications, the liver's apolipoproteins can cause disease. The stressed liver produces C reactive protein, which is a measure of inflammation and is a risk factor for diabetes, insulin resistance and coronary artery disease.

The low-density small particle (LDL) is directly associated with coronary artery disease.

Is Dietary Fat Bad?

Many scientists have tried to prove that dietary saturated fat is unhealthy. (Siri-Tarino PW, et al. (2010). *Am J Clin Nutr*. 91(3):535-546; Micha R, Mozaffarian D (2010). *Lipids*. 45(10):893-905.) This area remains controversial, as recent studies suggest that dietary saturated fats do not raise the risk of heart disease.

A meta-analysis (a statistical technique for combining the results from multiple studies) of 21 studies encompassing 350,000 subjects for more than 20 years showed no association of saturated fats and coronary heart disease.

Thus, we are left with expert opinions ("Level IV data"—see the chapter on supplements.) The prevailing opinions recommend decreasing saturated fat in the diet and replacing them with unsaturated fats in order to raise HDL and lower LDL. Remember—it's the low-density LDL that causes vascular damage.

In the past, many studies replaced fat calories with carbohydrate calories, but this did not decrease the incidence of coronary artery disease. In this discussion, you need to keep in mind that the liver will convert all excess protein and carbohydrates to fat for storage—calories do count, and caloric restriction has always worked to prolong longevity.

The Ugly Fat

Trans fats increased the risk of coronary artery disease as found in the Nurses' Health Study, and are thus considered to be harmful. Trans fats raise LDL, lower HDL, and increase C reactive protein—an additional marker for coronary artery disease. These trans fats are fats created by heating vegetable oils in the presence of hydrogen gas. Trans fats have longer shelf lives and are ideal for frying fast foods. In June, 2015, the FDA decided to ban all man-made trans fats from the food supply. Measures of total cholesterol alone are of little value.

The Nurses' Health Studies, started in 1976 by Dr. Frank Speizer and in 1989 by Dr. Walter Willett, are long-term studies of the health of female nurses. The studies followed 121,700 female registered nurses since 1976 and 116,000 female nurses since 1989 to assess risk factors for cancer and cardiovascular disease.

Increased Risk of Coronary Artery Disease

HIGH SMALL-PARTICLE LDL

LOW HDL

HIGH C-REACTIVE PROTEIN

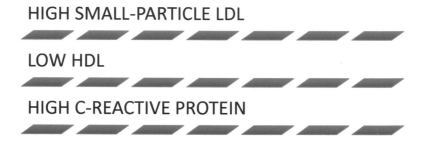

When Does Your Body Make Fat?

Your body makes fat whenever your body makes insulin. Thus, whenever you eat a meal, your blood glucose increases and your pancreas produces insulin to return your blood glucose level to normal. This is when your body makes fat.

Conversely, when you're asleep, you're fasting, and your body may consume fat as a source of energy.

The Value of Antioxidants

It is logical to expect that antioxidants would be beneficial, since they eliminate the free radicals or reactive oxygen species (ROS) that damage DNA and cause cell death. We are under constant attack from free radicals. They're in the air and the sunlight that hits our skin, and are produced whenever a cell generates energy from food. Free radicals steal electrons from other molecules and can damage cells and change metabolic processes.

Our bodies have developed molecules that donate electrons in order to neutralize free radicals, and these are "antioxidants." There are many types of antioxidants, and each is unique and acts in a specific situation; our bodies are continuously using them. Vitamin C, Vitamin E, Coenzyme Q10 are some examples; there are and hundreds more. Antioxidants are now being marketed just like fast food—all good, all of the time. Yet the antioxidants already present in our fruits and vegetables are sufficient to protect us from cell damage, and there is little evidence that increasing our intake through supplements is beneficial.

The antioxidant beta-carotene, when taken as a pill/supplement, actually increases the risk of lung cancer in smokers. (Albanes D (1999). *Am J Clin Nutr*. 69(6):1345-1350.) There is one exception, and that is in the prevention of the eye disease called macular degeneration, where an antioxidant mixture of beta-carotene, Vitamin E, Vitamin C and zinc was beneficial. (*AREDS Report No. 8* (2001), *Arch Opthalmol*. 119:1417-36.)

Reactive Oxygen Species and Mitochondria

Reactive oxygen species (ROS) are chemically-reactive molecules containing oxygen (one example is peroxide). ROS are involved in many biologic events occurring in both health and disease. Mitochondria are independent parts of the insides of cells, and they use oxygen and glucose to produce energy in the form of adenosine triphosphate (ATP).

Mitochondria are the "engines" inside cells, and ATP is the fuel for the cell. Mitochondria can divide when stimulated by energy demands, such as by exercise or work. There are discrete changes in the mitochondria of aging cells that contribute to the dysfunction seen in aging cells, especially the skeletal muscle cells. Mitochondria produce ROS as a signal to the cells that oxygen is limited, and the ROS induce responses to save the cells. In this situation, ROS are good.

Older mitochondria may become dysfunctional and produce excess ROS which cause problems and predispose one to metabolic syndromes. ROS are produced by the activated cells of the cellular immune system (when antigenic peptides are presented to T lymphocytes). T cells or T lymphocytes are a type of lymphocyte (a type of white blood cell) that plays a central role in cell-mediated immunity. A peptide antigen is the use of a peptide to trigger the immune system to develop antibodies to that peptide. Peptides are short strings of amino acids; longer chains are known as proteins.

ROS are then produced as part of the inflammatory response.

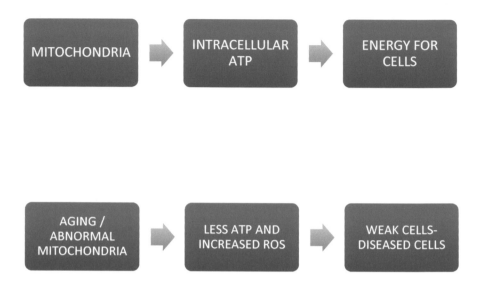

Skeletal muscle produces ROS during contraction in hypoxic (low oxygen) conditions. Excess ROS can damage skeletal muscle, and are implicated in the loss of muscle cells in immobilized muscle and underutilized muscle. ROS are implicated in age-related diseases and cancer.

To combat the overproduction of ROS, cells produce antioxidants such as thioredoxin and glutathione. (Droge W (2002). Physiol Rev. 82(1):47-95.)

In diabetes and obesity, there is a chronic excess of extracellular glucose and fatty acids producing excess ROS, causing insulin resistance and lipid deposition in the liver, heart and pancreas. ROS have a role in insulin resistance. (Summers SA, et al. (2005). *Diabetes*. 54(3):591-602.)

CHAPTER 4
DIET

What to Eat

The next question is "what to eat?" The answer depends on your goals. There's a difference between sports that require the participants to perform an action (such as gymnastics) and sports that are purely aesthetic (such as bodybuilding). There's also a difference between endurance sports (such as marathon running), speed sports (such as speed skating) and strength sports (such as weightlifting). Some wish to build muscle, lose body fat, increase energy level, and/or appear physically younger. The two most important principals are: (1) you must know what's healthy for you to eat; and (2) you must be in control of what you eat.

In order to be in control of what you eat, you must measure it. If you measure it, you can control it. I recommend an accurate scale and a daily written or electronic journal. The journal should contain a daily record of your weight, waist size, exercise activity, and quantitative food choices.

Body weight does not distinguish between muscle weight and fat weight. Measuring your waist size can be helpful as a measure of visceral body fat. Most people don't have regular access to the more accurate methods of measuring body fat, such as DEXA scans or Bod Pods (a machine that measures body mass when you sit inside of it).

The use of electrical impedance can be helpful, but only the expensive equipment is accurate. Simple skin calipers that measure skin thickness (subcutaneous fat) can be helpful, but don't measure visceral body fat.

I recommend taking a simple photograph of your body every week with your mobile phone and use the "BOD Keeper" app. The photo should be dated and kept with your other records. Using your computer, iPad or other tablet, or mobile phone for your recordkeeping is best. This will help to measure your progress and provide motivation to continue along your path.

According to research conducted by Fitbit, seeing an unflattering photographic image is a powerful source of motivation for losing weight. It certainly was for me!

The "best diet" is controversial, and the important aspect of food choice is that it achieves your goals and keeps you on a healthy path for life—one small step at a time. You need to ask yourself each week, "Am I better today than I was last week?" The answer should be, "Yes, I'm better—and I can prove it." Your journal will provide a behavior pattern that will help you to be successful in achieving your goals.

There should be no time pressure. Your path is comprised of small steps in the right direction. You've likely been "bad" for 20 or more years, and this can't be corrected in just weeks or months. Remember— this is a race won by the turtle.

The number of meals one should eat per day depends on your work requirements and lifestyle, and is a very controversial subject. There is no "best number of meals."

My recommended dietary preferences are based on science, tradition and common sense. The science is that of the Paleolithic diet that includes food choices of our early ancestors and excludes most milk products, most grains, and processed foods. (Eaton SB, et al. (1985). *N*

Engl J Med. 312:283-289.) Followers of this Paleolithic diet since childhood do not get obese nor get diabetes, hypertension, coronary artery disease or stroke. (Lindeberg S (2005). *Scand J Food Nutr*. 49:75-77.)

The non-scientific, traditional aspect of my diet mimics the diet recommended for bodybuilders, since my goal is to build muscle and decrease body fat. Not all aspects of the traditional bodybuilding diet have been scientifically tested, but the results are visible at competitions.

The common sense part of the diet is, "if it works, continue; if it doesn't work, change something."

If you like, you can skip the scientific part of this discussion and go straight to the list of healthy foods and the quick diet method.

Calories Count in the Beginning

In order to lose weight, you must take in fewer calories than your body needs to maintain your weight. This is carved in stone. With regard to simple weight loss, macronutrients don't matter. It doesn't matter whether it's high or low-carbohydrate, high or low-protein, or high or low-fat—as long as the total calories are below your needs. (Sacks FM, et al. (2009). *N Eng J Med*. 360:859-873.)

Macronutrients are important in determining which tissues you lose—muscle, fat or bone density—as well as what energy level you will have.

Intelligent Caloric Restriction

One interesting observation is that in many species, including primates—human beings, apes and monkeys—caloric restriction increases longevity. (Sinclair DA (2005). *Mechanisms of Aging and Development*. 126 (9):987-1002; Roth, et al. (2004). *J Science*. 305:1423-1426.) One theory to explain this phenomenon is that with fewer calories but sufficient essential minerals, amino acids and vitamins (thus, no malnutrition), there is less "oxidative stress" on the mitochondria in muscle cells. (Gredilla R, Batja G. Endocrine Society.

Published online 7/01/2013.) Mitochondria are small structures inside all living human cells that produce energy for cells. The analogy is that mitochondria are like the batteries that run the cell. Less oxidative stress means less damage to the DNA in the cells' mitochondria, leading to healthier muscle cells.

Your heart is a very important muscle, and cardiovascular disease remains the leading cause of death today. Perhaps we all need to lower

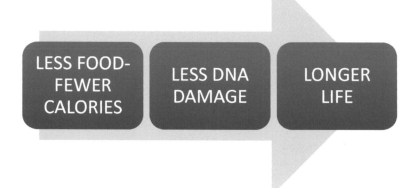

our calorie intake? A simple view of longevity is "the tennis ball theory" of life. The more the tennis ball (you) is hit over the net (stress), the less fuzz is left on it (decreased health).

We have only three variables that we can control with regard to our health: diet/food, activity/exercise, and supplements/medicines. According to the American Diabetes Association report of June, 2014, 29.3 million Americans, or 9.3% of the U.S. population, have diabetes. In seniors over 65 years of age, 25.9% were diabetic. Medical complications of diabetes include high blood pressure, abnormal lipids, heart disease, stroke, blindness, kidney disease and amputations. The total cost of diabetes to U.S. taxpayers in 2012 was approximately $245 billion. Much of this could have been saved by lifestyle changes including diet, exercise, supplements and medication.

It's not just a problem in the U.S., either. According to the World Health Organization in 2014, the global incidence of diabetes in adults over 18 years of age was 9%.

Fasting and Ketosis

Fasting is a behavior during which no calories are ingested. It may cause a state of "ketosis," where stored fats are broken down for energy, resulting in a build-up of acids called "ketones" within the body if prolonged). Fasting is part of many religious practices, and it has some beneficial effects. The Ramadan fast is intermittent, occurring only from sunrise to sunset, and ketosis does not usually occur, nor is there any change in athletic performance. (Chaouachi A, et al. (2012). *J Sports Sci.* 30(1):53-73.)

The ketogenic diet and ketosis were first studied scientifically by Vilhjalmur Stefansson and Eugene F. DuBois at Bellevue Hospital as a possible medical treatment. (Freeman JM, et al. (2007). *Pediatrics.* 119(3):535-543.) There are suggestions that a ketogenic diet may help epilepsy, obesity and diabetes.

If you eat few carbohydrates—fewer than 20 grams/day—your glucose reserves become depleted after two to three days. (Paoli A, et al. (2015). *Exerc Sports Sci Rev.* 43(3):153-162.) Ketone bodies are produced in this low-glucose environment to maintain energy levels, and are used as an energy source. Ketone bodies produce more energy than does glucose, due to greater mitochondrial ATP (adenosine triphosphate) production. Protein in the diet limits the use of amino acids as a glucose source, and increases satiety. Body fat decreases owing to increased lipid oxidation and decreased body fat production. In muscle cells, the mTOR (mechanistic target of rapamycin—an enzyme that regulates cell growth and division in response to energy levels, growth signals and nutrients) signaling is decreased, and this limits muscle growth. (Sandri M, et al. (2013). *Biogerontology.* 14(3):303-323.)

In summary, a very low-carbohydrate diet will help you lose body fat, *but* you will not be able to build muscle. You may experience greater fatigue initially. It's possible for your body to function normally, as well. However, muscle building will not occur.

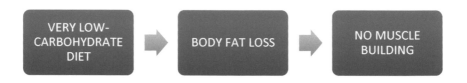

How Many Meals Per Day are Best?

Bodybuilders and many other athletes and dieters frequently eat a small meal every three to four hours. The thinking is that smaller meals increase the metabolic rate, lower insulin peaks, reduce hunger and lessen the risk of going off the diet. However, in controlled feeding studies, there was no significant difference between three meals per day and more than three meals per day. (Leidy HJ, Campbell WC (2011). *J Nutr*. 141(1):154-157.)

Fewer than three meals per day did result in an increase in perceived appetite and hunger, along with less appetite control. DO NOT SKIP BREAKFAST.

Resting Energy Expenditure (REE)

My diet starts at an arbitrary point based on resting energy expenditure (REE), with the expectation that this starting point will change. The units of the diet are calories, and this is for convenience. We will calculate a total daily calorie intake based on REE, and modify this based on activity level. (Mifflin MD, et al. (1990). Am J Clin Nutr. 51(2):241-247.)

Men:

10 x Weight(kg) + 6.25 x Height(cm) − 5 x Age (years) + 5.

Women:

10 x Weight(kg) + 6.25 x Height(cm) − 5 x Age (years) −161.

Please visit www.calorieline.com/tools/tdee; this site will calculate your REE for you.

We now modify this number by multiplying activity level:

No exercise = REE x 1.2

Active 3 days/week = REE x 1.375

Very active 3 days/week = REE x 1.55

Very active 5 days/week = REE x 1.725

Very active 7 days/week = REE x 1.9

A 40-year-old male, height 5'10", weighing 160 pounds, who is active three to five days/week, will need 2,545 calories per day to maintain his weight, and 2,045 calories per day to lose one pound per week. This is a precise number to be used as a starting point only, and should be altered when results do not occur.

We are not ready to eat just yet, since we still need to determine the *proportions* of the macronutrients—protein, carbohydrates and fat. Again this is another discrete value, and will need modification if it does not work. Since our presumed goal is building muscle and losing body fat, we will need approximately 30-40% of our calories as proteins, 30-50% carbohydrates, and 20-40% fats.

If you're pear-shaped (thick endomorph), you will need 40% protein, 20% carbohydrates and 40% fats. If you're a muscular athletic (mesomorph), you will need 40% protein, 30% carbohydrates and 30% fats. If you're thin and lean (ectomorph), you'll need 35% protein, 25% carbohydrates and 40% fats.

I suggest starting with 35% protein, 30% carbohydrates and 35% fats, for convenience only.

Now, with a calorie goal and macronutrient proportions, we can pick food groups.

- Daily Protein:
  2,045 calories x 35% = 716 calories.
  4 calories per gram of protein.
  716 ÷ 4 = 179 grams of protein per day;

- Daily Carbohydrates:

  2,045 calories x 30% = 613 calories.

  4 calories per gram of carbohydrates.

  715 ÷ 4 = 153 grams of carbohydrates per day.

- Daily Fat:

  2,045 calories x 35% = 716 calories.

  9 calories per gram of fat.

  716 ÷ 9 = 80 grams of fat per day.

Thus, a 40-year-old male, height 5' 10", weighing 160 pounds, who is active three to five days/week, will need 2,045 calories per day to lose one pound per week and build muscle, and he will eat 179 grams of protein, 153 grams of carbohydrate, and 80 grams of fat every day.

How many meals per day are optimal to build muscle and lose body fat? This has been discussed, and three or more meals per day will work. The important points: Eat when you're hungry; never skip a meal, since you won't be able to control your appetite; stop eating when nearly full—*never* overeat; always include a protein source in your meals to maintain satiety and to build muscle; and avoid eating for four hours prior to bedtime. However, if you awaken early and are hungry, please *do* eat, since you don't want muscle cells to be used as your energy source. Sleep is essential to decreasing cortisol levels and maintaining adequate leptin levels.

I suggest four to five meals per day in order to maintain a high-protein diet. Drink two liters of liquid per day, or enough liquid to keep your urine colorless.

Here are five sample meals containing approximately 500 calories per meal ("p/c/f/cal." = protein, carbohydrates, fat, calories):

- ½ cup of old-fashioned oatmeal made with water

  p/c/f/cal. = 5/27/3/150

  5 eggs

  p/c/f/cal. = 31/0.6/20/370

  ½ cup blueberries

  p/c/f/cal. = 0.5/10/0.25/40

- 7 oz. salmon
  p/c/f/cal. = 40/0/7.6/240
  2 whole-wheat pita p/c/f/cal.= 8/48/2/240
  salad as desired

- 6 oz. skinless chicken breast
  p/c/f/cal. = 52/0/6/280
  200 grams peeled yam
  p/c/f/cal. = 3/48/0.2/206
  Salad as desired

- 5 oz. broiled sirloin steak
  p/c/f/cal. = 43/0/10/285
  200 grams baked potato with skin
  p/c/f/cal. = 4.6/51/0.2/210
  salad as desired

- 8 oz. codfish
  p/c/f/cal. = 50/0/2/218
  195 grams long-grain brown rice
  p/c/f/cal. = 5/45/1.7/216
  Salad as desired

Now, please forget the above data collection and keep your own electronic or paper diary and measure your results. If you're losing inches from your waist, or one pound per week, you're doing well and should continue eating "healthy food" without all the precise measurements.

If all goes well, you should eat anything you desire one day a week— yes—one day of no restrictions! During this free day, healthy carbohydrates will increase your leptin levels and increase your metabolic rate (REE), since your body has been losing fat. Fat loss tends to lower leptin levels and REE. In order to maintain REE while building muscle and losing body fat, you must have an intense exercise program that raises your hormone levels. Supplements also become important.

Yes, we're attempting to change your body—you can lose body fat and build muscles at *any* age.

The Quick Diet

A simple method to help create a diet plan is to go to the Mayo Clinic calorie calculator (www.mayoclinic.org/calorie-calculator/itt-20084939) to calculate your daily calorie needs. This is your resting energy expenditure (REE)—the amount of calories your body uses every day.

Now subtract 500 calories from this number to determine your one-pound-per-week daily diet calories. Since our goal is to build muscle, we need 1-1.5 grams of protein per pound of body weight. Since protein in nature is always accompanied by fat, you'll have sufficient fat, as well. Thus, weigh your protein and calculate the calories using the MyFitnessPal app or website. Subtract the protein calories from your diet calories, and the remaining calories are available for carbohydrates. The MyFitnessPal.com website (not the mobile app) is excellent for finding the macronutrient and calorie content of most foods.

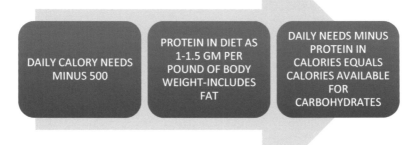

The Quick Formula for Protein, Fat and Carbohydrates in Your Diet

Quick Diet Formula—Example

(Mayo Clinic Calories – 500) minus (calorie content of 1.5 x body weight in pounds of protein choices) = calories available for carbohydrates. Thus, a 40-year-old male, weight 160 pounds, who is active three to five days/week, will need 2,045 calories per day to lose one pound per week and build muscle (179 grams of protein per day).

(Six large 2 ounce eggs = 36 grams of protein and 426 calories; 6 ounces of Atlantic wild salmon = 38 grams of protein and 348 calories; 8 ounces of chicken breast = 50 grams of protein and 240 calories; 8 ounces of lean steak = 48 grams of protein and 400 calories.)

The above four protein meals total approximately 172 grams of protein and 1,414 total protein and fat calories. This leaves 2,045 — 1,414 = 631 calories remaining for carbohydrates.

This is a good place to start. Protein shakes made from whey protein and low in carbohydrates can be substituted for a meal. Remember—as long as you're moving in the direction of your goals, you're doing well. If you plateau—and you will!—you just need to change something. The only things *you* control are your food choices and your exercise program.

In my personal diet, when preparing for a bodybuilding competition, I always plateau at some point. When I plateau, I just eliminate anything that will block leptin—gluten, MSG and artificial sweeteners. Since insulin is the major leptin blocker, I increase my fiber with salads, and limit my intermediate/high-glycemic carbohydrates to small servings of oatmeal, yams and rice. If this doesn't work, then I limit my protein sources to fish, skinless white-meat chicken, and protein shakes with whey from New Zealand. I also "move more and eat less."

This diet isn't a specific diet for all readers, but rather outlines a simple method of finding a starting point for anyone's diet when knowing only calorie count and protein requirements.

We All Need to be Athletes: Protein From Food

We've discussed the essential role of protein in your body. To summarize, protein is essential to build and repair your tissues. Athletes need a high-protein diet. (Tipton KD, Wolf RR (2004). *J Sport Sc.* 22(1):65-79.) For us to remain healthy, we need to exercise and be "athletes," and try to eat 1 gram of protein per pound of body weight. Bodybuilders need up to 3.6 grams per pound, and possibly more. (Lemon PW (2000). *J Am College of Nutr.* 19(85):513S-21S.)

Healthy protein foods include whole eggs, Egg Beaters, fish, shellfish, skinless chicken, skinless turkey, lean beef, lean lamb, lean pork loin, unflavored Greek yogurt and low-fat cottage cheese. Protein is also available from vegetable sources, such as legumes, broccoli, peas, nuts and spinach. There is a measurable decrease in total testosterone production in athletes eating a vegetable protein diet compared to athletes who eat proteins from animal sources. This decrease occurred after just six weeks. (Rabin A, et al. (1992). *Med Sci Sports Exerc.* 24(11):1290-1297.)

Protein Supplements

Protein supplements are powders or premixed powders made from milk, eggs or plants. The most popular protein supplement is whey protein made from milk. Whey protein is rapidly absorbed. If lactose intolerance is a concern, lactose-free whey protein is also available in the form of whey isolate or whey hydrolysate.

Casein protein is also made from milk, and is more slowly absorbed than whey. Egg protein is absorbed even more slowly. Egg and whey protein supplements are equal in their ability to stimulate muscle growth in animals. (Norton LE, et al. (2012). *Nutrition and Metabolism.* 9(1):67.)

Soy protein is controversial. The Harvard School of Public Health, as of February, 2014, gives soy protein mixed reviews—their "Straight Talk" is not so straight. The concerns regarding the estrogen-like isoflavones in soy protein is still a topic of research. Much depends upon the amount of soy protein in your diet, and how your gastrointestinal bacteria help to metabolize isoflavones. (Cara L, et al. (2005). *Br J Nutr.* 94(6):873-876.) Other noncontroversial plant-based protein supplements are available, with pea proteins being the best quality.

Fat in Your Food: The Media, Politics and Bad Science of Heart Disease—Who Controls Cultural Knowledge?

The most tragic story regarding health during the last 65 years is the high incidence in coronary artery disease in the U.S. Doctors today expect patients, as they age, to have some coronary artery disease and high blood pressure. Your heart is mostly muscle tissue that works continuously. Coronary artery disease occurs when the coronary arteries that supply your heart muscles accumulate fatty plaques that impede blood flow to the muscle. When blood flow stops, the muscle area involved dies, and this is called a "heart attack" or "myocardial infarction." When your heart muscles are starved for blood, you get chest pain called "angina." When your weakened heart muscles cannot pump blood out of the heart, you become short of breath and can go into "congestive heart failure."

According to the Centers for Disease Control and Prevention, 610,000 people die of heart disease in the U.S. every year—that's one in every four deaths. (CDC, NCHS. *Underlying Cause of Death 1999-2013* on CDC WONDER Online Database, released 2015. Data is from the *Multiple Cause of Death Files*, 1999-2013, as compiled from data provided by the 57 vital statistics jurisdictions through the Vital Statistics Cooperative Program. Accessed Feb. 3, 2015.)

Heart disease is the leading cause of death for both men and women. More than half of deaths due to heart disease in 2009 were in men. Coronary heart disease is the most common type of heart disease, killing over 370,000 people annually. Every year, about 735,000 Americans have a heart attack. Of these, 525,000 are a first heart attack, and 210,000 happen in people who have already had a heart attack. (Mozaffarian D, Benjamin EJ, Go AS, et al. (2015). *Circulation.* 131:e29-322.)

Some of the blame for these deaths can be attributed to bad science, politics, and the media. Public opinion and public behavior can be the measures of our "cultural knowledge," and from the 1950s to the present, our cultural knowledge blamed cholesterol, red meat and saturated fat in the diet for causing the increase in heart disease. This thinking was inaccurate, and only recently has the truth emerged that the blame belongs on trans fats, carbohydrates and insulin resistance.

The incorrect thinking was as follows: fat in the diet causes fat to accumulate in the arteries that supply the muscles of the heart. The arteries get clogged—much like the drain in a sink—and some heart muscle dies.

There is no science to support this simple theory. The result of this "bad science" was dietary recommendations that actually increased the incidence of coronary artery disease from approximately 1960 to 2014 by recommending a high-carbohydrate diet. During these years, both the American Heart Association (AHA) and the U.S. Department of Agriculture (USDA) recommended a diet minimizing meat products and maximizing carbohydrates—fruits, vegetables and whole grains. On January 1, 2012, Mark Bittman, a *New York Times* columnist, wrote, "...to eat better...the answer is known to everyone...eat more plants." On November 4, 1993, there was a television episode of *Seinfeld* with Mayor Rudy Giuliani regarding the "horrors" of finding fat in the non-fat yogurt. Even at the time of this writing, National Public Radio, on 7/25/15, featured the new Surgeon General of the U.S., Vivek Murthy, who reminded people to eat fruits and vegetables—no mention was made of protein or fat—just carbohydrates.

The demonization of dietary animal fats/saturated fats finds its origins in the work of Ancel Benjamin Keys. He, and others, found that cholesterol was the main ingredient in the blocked areas of the coronary arteries. (Keys A (1953 Nov). *Am J Public Health Nations Health.* 43(11):1399-1407.)

The idea that a low-fat, low-cholesterol diet would prove to prevent heart disease seems reasonably logical, but has never been scientifically proven in ethnographic population studies nor in prospective studies.

Current evidence does not clearly support cardiovascular guidelines that encourage high consumption of polyunsaturated fatty acids and low consumption of total saturated fats. (Chawdhury R, et al. (2014). *Annals Int Med.* 160(6):398-406.) It is very difficult today to do large population prospective studies, for a variety of reasons: it's difficult to control human dietary choices; it's difficult to prevent changes in diet over time; and it's difficult to define low-fat and high-fat diets in different countries. The famous Mediterranean diet had all of these problems, yet concluded that there is something favorably affecting the lower incidence of coronary artery disease in the Mediterranean populations of Greece and Italy. (Dontas AS, et al. (2008). *Clin Interv Aging*. 3(2):397.)

Approximately 50 years ago, Keys and colleagues described strikingly low rates of coronary heart disease in the Mediterranean region, where fat intake was relatively high but largely from olive oil. Controlled feeding of high-cholesterol and high-fat diets has shown that compared to carbohydrates, both monounsaturated and polyunsaturated fats reduce LDL and triglycerides and increase HDL cholesterol—thus being beneficial and contrary to what Keys predicted. (Willett WC (2006 Feb). *Public Health Nutr*. 9(1A):105-10.)

The Nurses' Health Study of 78,788 women clearly demonstrated that trans fat from partially hydrogenated vegetable oils (absent in traditional Mediterranean diets) was most strongly related to the risk of coronary artery disease. Polyunsaturated and monounsaturated fat were inversely associated with risk and were thus healthy. (Oh K, et al. (4/1/2005). *Am J Epidemiol*. 161(7):672-9.)

Why dietary fat is rarely mentioned in the media as beneficial, despite objective scientific studies, remains a mystery. Who controls our cultural knowledge?

Accurate dietary population studies have been conducted in a 10,000-square-mile area of Kenya and Tanzania, where the Maasai tribe lives. The Maasai have few dietary choices, and their regular diet is 66% fat and consists almost entirely of cow's blood, milk and meat. Their serum cholesterol and beta-lipoprotein levels are low. The proof of the principle is that post-mortem dissection of their coronary arteries shows almost no coronary artery disease, and electrocardiograms (EKG or ECG) of the men show no evidence of old heart attacks (myocardial infarctions). (Biss K, et al. (1971). *NEJM*. 284:1284-1304.)

An important additional finding was that Maasai men weigh less and have lower blood pressure levels than American and European men. The Maasai have body weights and blood pressure levels that remain nearly constant as they age, unlike American men, who nearly always gain weight and have higher blood pressure as they age.

Healthy fats consist of whole eggs, tree nuts, olive oil, seeds, nut oils, avocados and ground tree-nut butter and peanut butter. Avoid commercial nut butters that have added sugar.

The saturated fat present in meat and dairy products is essential and healthy, as well. However, the total calorie content of your diet is still a limiting factor in food choices. For this reason, it's important to trim visible fat from red meat, buy low-fat ground beef, remove the skin from poultry, and purchase low-fat dairy products such as low-fat cottage cheese and unflavored Greek yogurt. Please avoid drinking milk, since it is unusually insulinogenic, and the calories do count.

Carbohydrates in Your Diet

Healthy carbohydrates include all vegetables, all berries, other fruits (with the exception of bananas, grapes, figs and dates, which contain too much sugar relative to fiber), old-fashioned oatmeal, beans (garbanzo, kidney, navy, pinto and black), and yams. A small amount of rice eaten with protein is healthy, despite being a high-glycemic carbohydrate.

It is important to have vegetables or salads as often as you like— every day—to ensure sufficient fiber.

Unhealthy carbohydrates have a high glycemic index, meaning they raise blood glucose levels quickly and so raise insulin levels quickly, and therefore produce body fat quickly. Examples include any food with added sugar, soft drinks, fruit juice, any juice, pasta, pancakes, waffles, bread, pastry, cake, pie, cookies, ice cream, sorbet, candy, and most cold cereals. We've already discussed the glycemic index earlier in this book.

Carbohydrates and insulin are also essential for your body. Insulin is necessary for storing glycogen in your liver and in muscle cells, in addition to storing fat in fat cells. All of your cells need energy from sugar. This is where calories count, and we get fat and unhealthy only when we consume more calories than we burn.

In the presence of adequate protein, low-carbohydrate diets and high-carbohydrate diets give similar weight loss results. (Johnston CS, et al. (2006). *Am J Clin Nutr.* 83(5):1055-1061.) Muscle growth improves in the presence of insulin. (Gelfand RA, Barrett EJ (1987). *J Clin Invest.*

80(1):1-6.)

Very low-carbohydrate diets raise serum cortisol levels and lower testosterone levels, resulting in fatigue and less muscle growth. (Lane AR, et al. (2010). *Euro J Appl Physiol.* 108(6):1125-1131.)

The question of what is the best amount of carbohydrates for your diet has been discussed earlier, and the amount will vary based on your goals, body shape (% body fat), and exercise intensity. *You need carbohydrates.*

Foods Best Avoided

You shouldn't eat any man-made wheat products, nor any food when you don't know its ingredients.

Alcohol

Alcohol can have positive health benefits when consumed in moderation, and negative health benefits when consumed in excess. The line between these two situations is very precise in research. Moderate alcohol intake decreases the risk of coronary artery disease by 40-70%, according to multiple prospective studies. (O'Keefe JH, et al. (2007). *Am Coll Cardiol.* 50:1009.) (This is Level III data—please refer to the Supplements section of this book, where levels of evidence are explained.)

These studies were not randomized, and had different definitions of a "standard drink." The studies did pass a meta-analysis—a statistical analysis of 34 separate studies. The conclusion of these 34 studies, involving over 1 million subjects, was that alcohol drinkers have a lower risk of dying from a heart attack. A standard drink in the U.S. is 14-15 grams of alcohol. This could be 12 ounces of beer, 5 ounces of wine, or 1.5 ounces of 80 proof liquor. More than two standard drinks per day in women and three drinks per day in men, however, did increase the risk of dying.

Similar results have been found with regard to peripheral vascular disease and stroke. Stroke is an event wherein the blood supply to a part of the brain is occluded, and brain cells die.

The "French paradox" refers to the low incidence of coronary artery mortality in a country with a high incidence of smoking and high consumption of saturated fat. The theory to explain France's lower-than-expected coronary heart disease was the high consumption of red wine. (Renaud S, de Longeril M (1992). *Lancet*. 339:1523.)

Other studies do not confirm any specific alcoholic beverage type as being better for coronary artery health, but all studies show that the amount of alcohol is important. In summary, moderate alcohol consumption—defined as two standard drinks per day for men—lowers HDL C, triglycerides, C reactive protein, platelet aggregation and fibrinogen levels, and would be expected to lower a person's risk of coronary heart disease by nearly 25%. (Rimm EB, et al. (1999). *BMJ*. 319:1523-1528.)

Achieving a balance between the health risks and benefits of alcohol consumption remains difficult, as each person has a different susceptibility to the adverse health consequences associated with alcohol consumption—addiction, dementia, cirrhosis, hypertension, diabetes, cardiomyopathy, congestive heart failure, and bone marrow suppression. Among participants aged 30 to 59 years and free of hypertension, diabetes and cardiovascular disease, the lowest death rate was found with consumption of less than one drink daily. Conversely, among participants aged 60 to 79 years and with one of the aforementioned conditions, the lowest death rate occurred with a consumption of three drinks per day.

Misunderstood Foods

The least understood and most controversial food is saturated fat—the fat found in dairy and red meat. Over the years, data has revealed that dietary saturated fatty acids (saturated fats) are *not* associated with coronary artery disease.

Smoothies are smooth because the fiber has been broken down, and are thus not as healthy as the original ingredients when eaten individually. Juice is just sugar—glucose and fructose—along with water and some vitamins. It's best to take a multivitamin and avoid the sugar.

Artificial sweeteners are not well understood. If you believe in Pavlov, diet soda should be bad for you—but I will admit that I still drink an occasional Diet Coke. With artificial sweeteners, your brain senses sugar and the pancreas releases insulin. (Pepino MY, et al. (Sept. 2013). *Diabetes Care.* 36(9):2530-2535.) You already know that higher insulin levels create more body fat and can lead to leptin resistance.

Despite what critics say, caffeine can be healthy. Early studies showing coffee as harmful were done when the harmful effects of smoking were not taken into consideration, and most coffee drinkers in the past also smoked cigarettes.

According to the Mayo Clinic, coffee may protect you from Parkinson's disease, diabetes and liver cancer. Coffee improves cognitive function and memory, and decreases the risk of depression by blocking the inhibitory neurotransmitter adenosine. (Fredholm BB (1995). *Pharmacology and Toxicology.* 76(2):93-101.)

Caffeine is a "fat burner," and can increase adrenaline levels and release fatty acids from the fat tissues. Coffee can increase your metabolic rate by 3-11%. (Dilloo AG, et al. (1989). *Am J Clin Nutr.* 49 (10):44-50.)

A cup of coffee can improve your performance in the gym by 11-12%. (Doherty M, Smith PM (2004). *Int J Sport Nutr Exerc Metab.* 6:626-646.)

Milk has an unusually high insulin response that is greater than predicted by its carbohydrate and protein content. Most milk products should be avoided, the exceptions being unflavored yogurt and low-fat cottage cheese. (Ostman EM, et al. (2001). *Am J Clin Nutr.* 74(1):96-100.)

Not all fruits are healthy. Fruit contains fructose, which can only be metabolized by the liver. This can lead to metabolic syndrome. If enough fiber is present—such as in berries—the damage is less. Bananas, dates, grapes and figs have excessive fructose and glucose, and contain insufficient fiber, and thus should be avoided.

Wheat products should be avoided—bread, most cold cereals, and pasta. Wheat products are high-glycemic carbohydrates and by themselves raise insulin levels. All wheat products also contain gluten.

Gluten is a vegetable protein that is difficult for your body to digest. The problem with gluten is not the rare gluten sensitivity, but rather that gluten blocks the activity of leptin. Leptin, as you may recall, is released by fat cells and tells your body to burn fat and stop eating. Known leptin blockers include insulin, artificial sweeteners, gluten, and the seasoning monosodium glutamate (MSG).

Eat all the vegetables and salads that you like. The energy required to metabolize and digest salads and vegetables equals the added calories. The fiber is the real value of salads and vegetables. The magic of fiber is its ability to slow absorption of all other foods in the mix, and decrease insulin levels.

There is no substitute for single-source real food that occurs in nature. When in doubt, read the label. Any box or can of food with a label contains processed products that do not occur normally in nature. "Heart healthy" may not be healthy for you, such as is the case of most boxed cereals.

Metabolic syndrome is a modern disease associated with man-made food. You've been raised on and have become accustomed to eating processed, man-made food. It's time to stop eating this stuff and restore your body to good health. Don't listen to the advertisements that market foods—*none* of these unnatural, man-made products are healthy.

CHAPTER 5
EXERCISE

The Benefits of Exercise, the Missing Ingredient: Metabolic Role of Exercise

We will define exercise, for our purposes, as physical activity requiring effort designed to improve health. Exercise can be designed to improve endurance, strength, balance and flexibility. Even a small amount of daily exercise will make you live longer. (Wen CP, et al. (2011). *Lancet*. 378:1244-1253.)

Exercise is the missing ingredient in most unhealthy lifestyles. It can reverse the metabolic syndrome. Epidemiological studies reveal a higher incidence of metabolic syndrome in people who don't exercise. (Rennie KL, et al. (2003). *J Epidemiol*. 32:600-606.) Supervised long-term, intense exercise raises high-density lipoprotein (HDL), lowers triglycerides and reduces blood pressure. Both diet and exercise are required to lower insulin resistance. (Carroll S, Dudfield M (2004). *Sports Med*. 34(6):371-418.)

Aerobic interval training is superior to continuous moderate exercise for enhancing endothelial function, improving insulin signaling, lowering blood glucose levels, and deceasing lipogenesis in adipose tissue. Both types of exercise are equally effective for lowering blood pressure and weight loss. (Tjonna AE, et al. (2008). *Circulation*. 118 (4):346-354.)

The benefits of exercise are observable inside the skeletal muscle cells, with an increase in the size and number of mitochondria. (Holloszy JO (2008). *J Physiol Pharmacol*. 59 Suppl. 7:5-18.)

Exercise builds muscle, and it's the *only* way one can build muscle. Aging and the associated decline in muscle capacity are associated with a decline in mitochondria content and function. A similar mitochondria decline is seen in insulin resistance and maturity onset diabetes. (Menshikova EV, et al. (2006). *J Gerontol A Biol Sci Med*. 61(6):534-540.) Exercise increases the number of mitochondria in cells, and these new mitochondria then burn more energy with greater efficiency. The cells in the liver produce less visceral fat. (Thuy S, et al. (2008). *J Nutr*. 138:1452-1455.)

Exercise decreases both glucose and insulin levels, and with proper diet, can reverse insulin resistance. Exercise will improve the brain's response to leptin and decrease cortisol levels. The best treatment for stress relief and insomnia is exercise.

There are two broad categories of exercise. Cardiovascular exercises (endurance training—ET) are aimed at improving the heart, lungs and circulation. Resistance training (RT) exercises are designed to strengthen and build muscles.

The American Heart Association recommends both ET and RT for both people with and without heart disease. (Williams MA, et al. (2007). *Circulation*. 116:572-584.) Both RT (weightlifting) and ET (running, swimming, jogging, biking) improve health, but each has different benefits.

With regard to body composition, both types of exercise increase bone mineral density and prevent bone loss and fracture. ET is better for increasing body fat loss, while RT increases muscle mass and strength, thus increasing lean body mass. Both are equally effective with regard to glucose metabolism, and insulin levels and sensitivity. Both are nearly equally effective for lipid control; ET has a slight advantage in lowering triglycerides. ET is clearly superior for cardiovascular dynamics—lower resting heart rate, cardiac output and cellular oxygen consumption (VO2 max). RT is better for increasing the basal metabolic rate. Both are equally effective for quality of life measures.

THE BENEFITS OF EXERCISE	REVERSES METABOLIC SYNDROME; INCREASES INSULIN SENSITIVITY; IMPROVED LEPTIN SIGNALLING
	RAISES GOOD HDL AND LOWERS TRYGLYCERIDES
	DECREASES BLOOD PRESSURE
	BUILDS MUSCLE AND INCREASES STRENGTH
	DECREASES STRESS
	PROLONGS LIFE
	REDUCED C-REACTIVE PROTEIN

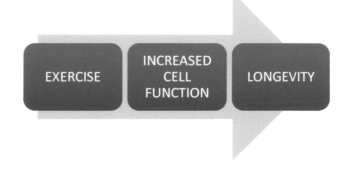

Both types of exercise are important. It's sad to see an obese person with a joint or bone injury that prevents their ability to exercise and limits their ability to prevent insulin resistance and subsequent metabolic syndrome.

Obese people have a high fracture rate. (Manias K, et al. (2006). *Bone*. 39:652-657.) The benefits of exercise are short-lived, and thus exercises must be done frequently and regularly in order to maintain their beneficial effects. Exercise will restore your cells to a higher level of health, with efficient mitochondria and increased function.

As mentioned previously, exercise and diet can eliminate metabolic syndrome. You now have the "basic scientific knowledge" of how your body works. Would you like to know more? Do you want to know how to look and feel younger?

How to be Strong, Robust and Healthy

In this chapter, we'll discuss what science can tell us about muscle building. The assumption is that muscle strength at any age increases your activity level and improves your quality of life. In the "tennis ball theory of life," the more the ball is hit over the net, the less fuzz is left on it. For our purposes, "hitting the ball" is analogous to the stresses of life, and the resulting reactive oxygen species (ROS) damage your DNA is "less fuzz."

So, how do we get more fuzz on the ball? We can do this by building more muscle with resistance exercises and by using the correct supplements and nutrients.

Exercise Will Lengthen Your Life and Improve Your Health

There is objective data indicating that exercise will lengthen your life span. (Mouaz H, et al. (2014). *Cl Cardiol*. 37 (8):456-461.) The data is positive for all age groups, with results being most pronounced in men over 60 years of age. Vigorous exercise is even more beneficial. (Lee IM, et al. (1995). *JAMA*. 273(15):1179-1184.) This may appear to be obvious and logical, but it was not objectively proven until 1995.

The information in this book introducing you to exercise and disseminating knowledge regarding the body is based on scientific data. By implementing your new-found knowledge, you'll be able to change the way you look and feel.

Exercise will affect, in some way, every cell in your body. Your body will change when stressed, and will adapt. This is referred to as Specific Adaption to the Imposed Demand (SAID). (*Oxford Dictionary of Sports Medicine* (1998). Michael Kent.) This is what exercise does. What form of exercise you choose will depend upon *you*—your abilities, your motivation, and your goals—*just you*.

Your body needs energy constantly, whether at rest or while exercising. We discussed this in the section on adenosine triphosphate (ATP) and mitochondria. The mitochondria are independent parts of the interior of cells, and they use oxygen and glucose to produce energy in the form of ATP.

Mitochondria are the "engines" inside cells. As mentioned earlier, when you increase your exercise, your muscle cells adapt by increasing the number of mitochondria and produce more ATP. When this occurs, you burn fat, and your muscles produce more force. You are now on your path to a healthy lifestyle.

In time, and with patience and the knowledge gained from this book, you'll begin reshaping your body by burning fat and increasing muscle mass. The force of your muscle contractions will strengthen your bones. The heart muscles will enlarge and become more efficient in order to pump more blood to your skeletal muscles. The number of small blood vessels throughout your body will increase throughout, and your brain will become more efficient. Your perceived stress, as measured by cortisol output, will decrease; you'll sleep better and will experience less anxiety and more energy; you will live longer. Exercise benefits every organ in your body.

Now that you want to exercise, how much and what type is best?

Mental Health and Exercise

According to the National Institute of Mental Health, in 2013, there were approximately 10 million adults aged 18 or older in the U.S. who had some form of serious mental illness (SMI). This represented 4.2% of all U.S. adults. (nimh.nih.gov.) A "serious mental illness" is defined as a mental, emotional or behavioral problem that results in impairment of lifestyle and meets the criteria specified in the *Diagnostic and Statistical Manual of Mental Disorders*.

In 2006, the Agency for Healthcare Research and Quality estimated the cost of SMI in the U.S. to be $57.5 billion due solely to the loss of income.

Depression is a common illness, affecting at least 1 in 5 people during their lifetime. Exercise has been advocated as an adjunct to the usual treatment. A review and meta-analysis done by Cochrane identified all available randomized trials which compared exercise with either no treatment or an established treatment. In 23 trials (907 participants) which compared exercise with no treatment or a control intervention, the data indicated a large clinical benefit. Exercise did seem to improve the symptoms of depression. (Mead GE, et al. (2009). *Cochrane Database of Systematic Reviews*, Issue 3. Art. No. CD004366. DOI: 10.1002/14651858. pub 4.)

The effects of aerobic and nonaerobic exercise on anxiety levels, absenteeism, job satisfaction and resting heart rate were investigated. Results indicated that aerobic subjects significantly reduced their anxiety levels over a single exercise session. Post-exercise anxiety decreased over eight weeks for both groups. There were no changes evident in job satisfaction, absenteeism or resting heart rate.

These results show that aerobic exercise is superior to nonaerobic exercise for anxiety reduction. (Altchiler L, Motta R (1994). *J Clin Psychol*. 50:829-840.)

Insomnia

Pharmacotherapy in the form of sleeping pills is the most oft-prescribed treatment for insomnia. However, sleep aids carry side effects and may not be recommended for long-term treatment. Exercise may, instead, prove to be the treatment of choice.

In one study, patients aged 50 to 76 years with moderate sleep complaints were randomized to either 16 weeks of moderate-intensity exercise training or a wait-listed control condition. Exercise consisted of four daily 30- to 40-minute periods of endurance training (low-impact aerobics or brisk walking) prescribed at 60% to 75% of maximal heart rate. Patients in the exercise group showed significant improvement in sleep parameters of self-rated sleep quality. (King AC, et al. (1997). *JAMA*. 277(1):32-37.)

How Much Exercise is Enough?

Cardiovascular exercises include running, jogging, swimming, cycling, elliptical, and using the newer cardiovascular equipment. The relative intensity of cardiovascular exercise is easily measured by two simultaneous methods: the subjective "talk test," and the objective measure of heart rate. It's easy to use a heart rate monitor, and many exercise devices have built-in heart monitors.

According to the Mayo Clinic, vigorous exercise occurs when your heart rate is 50% to 85% of your Maximum Heart Rate (MHR). This formula determines your MHR: 220 minus your age.

With vigorous activity, you won't be able to speak complete sentences due to being out of breath. This is a very simple definition of "vigorous," but it's a measurable starting point for most active adults. This method of MHR determination isn't accurate for athletes who have ventricular hypertrophy with a slow baseline heart rate.

A more complicated approach, as recommended by the National Academy of Sports Medicine, defines Target Heart Rate = (Maximum Heart Rate minus Resting Heart Rate) x Desired Intensity % + Resting Heart Rate. (Karvonen J, Vuorimaa T (1988). *Sports Medicine*. 5 (5):303-311.)

The Centers for Disease Control and Prevention recommend 150 minutes (2½ hours) per week of cardiovascular exercise such as brisk walking every week, as well as muscle-strengthening activities two to three days per week which address all major muscle groups. Another cardiovascular option is 75 minutes per week of vigorous exercise (such as jogging or running), again with two to three days per week of muscle-strengthening exercises.

Muscle building activities in general should involve weight or resistance training for each muscle group at least once a week. Each muscle should be exercised to failure once a week.

This training is the only path to increase the muscle mass that you're otherwise losing. Modern physical therapy science teaches us that before we can build muscle safely and efficiently, we must be flexible and have core strength.

High-Intensity Interval Training (HIIT)

High-intensity interval training is a type of endurance training involving short periods of maximal effort followed by periods of maintenance or recovery effort. What can differ is the timing and type of endurance exercise.

A typical cycling HIIT pattern may be four to six maximal (all-out) 30-second cycling sprints separated by four to five-minute recovery periods of comfortable cycling. When HIIT is compared to longer steady endurance training, the HIIT patterns show increased mitochondrial density in muscle cells and greater muscle performance improvements. (Gibala M (2009). *Applied Physiol Nutr Metab.* 34(4):428-432; Billat LV (2001). *Sports Med.* 31(1):13-31.)

Flexibility and Warm-Up; Myofascial Release; Dynamic Stretching

Warming up before and after exercising has been studied in detail. This area of study has many variables and is quite complex. "Flexibility" is defined as the ability of skeletal muscles and tendons to lengthen. Muscles and tendons are covered with soft tissue called "fascia" which provide tension and support. In response to injury or resistance training, fascia changes in tension and becomes less elastic. (Barnes MF (1997). J Bodywork and Movement Th. 1(4).) The fascia will limit flexibility and range of motion unless it's manually stretched. Thus, it's important to first release the fascia by way of myofascial release or massage before exercising the muscle.

Static flexibility measures the range of motion of a joint. An example of static stretching is bending to touch your toes. Static stretching before exercising will not prevent injury or soreness, and it will make the muscle transiently weaker. (Fowles JR, et al. (2000). *J Applied Physiology*. 89(3):1179-1188.)

However, static stretching a muscle for 30 seconds on a regular basis will increase the range of motion of the muscle, and this is an important benefit. (Bandy WD, Irion JM (2015). *Physical Therapy*. 95(4).)

The best time to perform static stretching is after the muscle has been exercised, *not* before. Static stretching is not a good "warm up."

Dynamic stretching is the ideal warm up. Dynamic stretching involves a repetitive joint movement that increases in range with each repetition and increases body temperature. It's important to increase the flow of blood to the tendons and muscles you're about to exercise. It's also important for your brain to activate as many of the muscles that are involved in this joint movement as possible. Examples of dynamic stretching include knee bends, jumping jacks and jogging. There are many testimonials from athletic coaches published in the *Journal of Strength and Conditioning* which support this type of warm up.

The big picture is that flexibility or increased range of motion will improve if you perform myofascial release followed by light dynamic stretching before exercising, and static stretching after you exercise. Myofascial release may also be beneficial after exercising.

Examples of Myofascial Release

WARM-UP ROUTINE BEFORE EXERCISE	MYOFASCIAL
	DYNAMIC STRETCH
	EXERCISE

Using Foam Roller; Dynamic Stretching

Releasing Piriformis and Gluteus

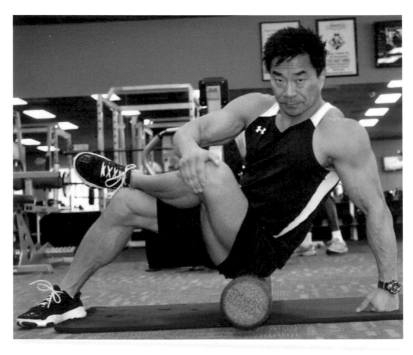

Myofascial Release Using Foam Roller:
Relaxing Iliotibial Band

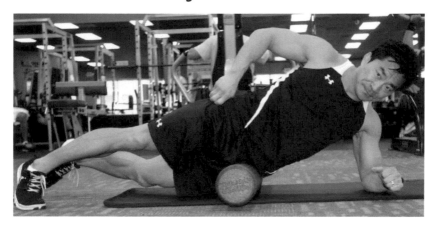

Releasing Adductors

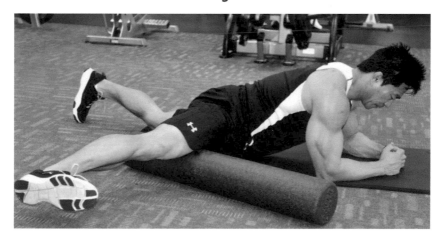

Myofascial Release Using Foam Roller:
Releasing Calves

Myofascial release is an important part of each training day, and can be done pre and post-exercise. It's an important part of any flexibility program, as well as exercise recovery programs.

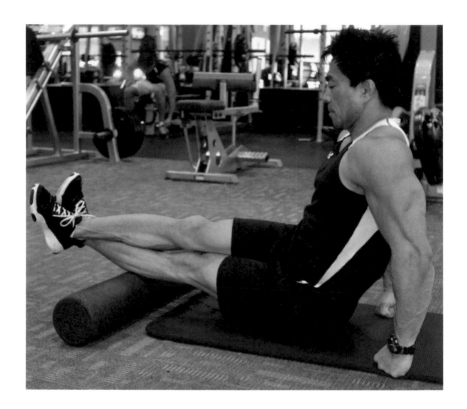

Releasing Latissimus Dorsi

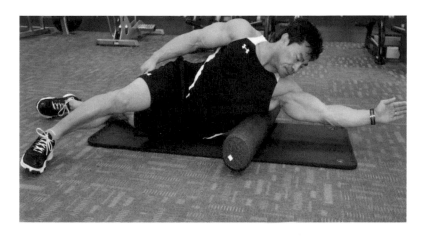

Releasing Erector Spinae

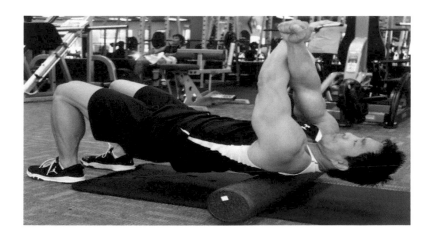

Dynamic Stretching:

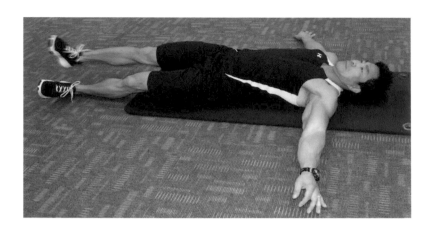

Repetitive Joint Movement

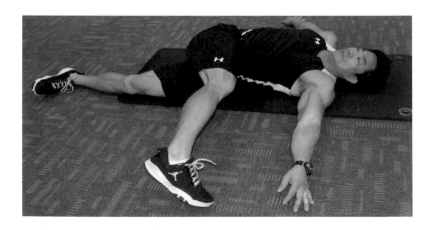

Dynamic Stretching

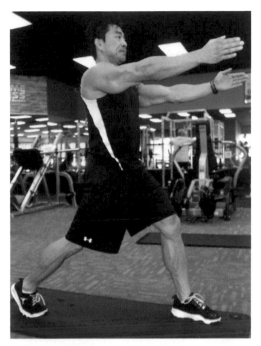

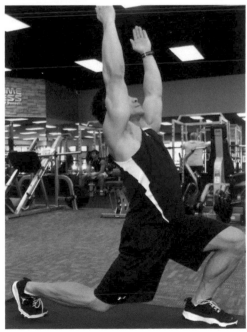

Dynamic Stretching

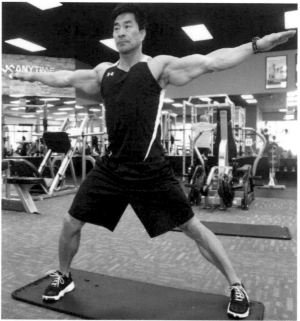

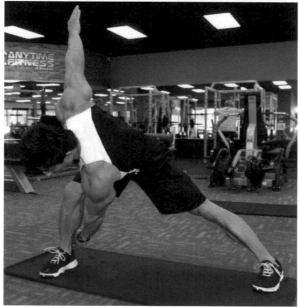

Dynamic Stretching

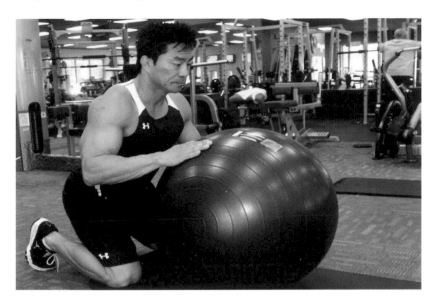

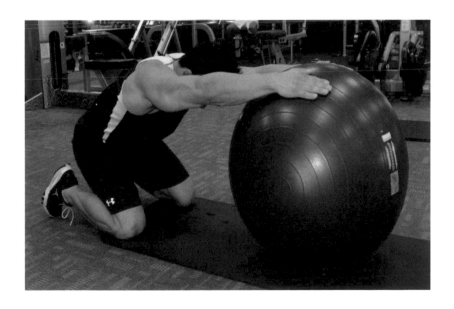

The Core—Your Most Important Muscles

The core muscles connect the arms and chest to the pelvis. Core muscles create stability between your upper and lower body when you perform complex movements, such as running, lifting and twisting. The core muscles align the spine, ribs and pelvis, and thus are the basis of one's posture. The major core muscles include the pelvic floor, the transverse abdominis, the internal and external obliques, the rectus abdominis, and all the muscles of the spine and buttocks.

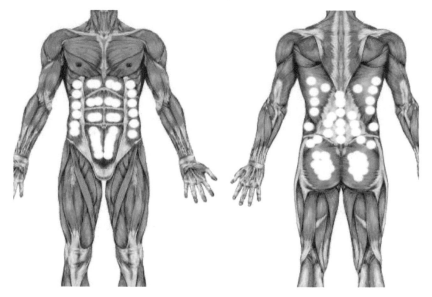

The above picture highlights some of the more visible anterior and posterior core muscles. Other internal core muscles, not visible above, are responsible for urinary and bowel continence.

Core muscles initiate all dynamic physical activities in nearly every sport. Many sports injuries, including those causing back pain, happen due to weak core muscles. Both yoga and Pilates improve core stability and can be a very important part of your exercise program.

Examples of Core Exercises

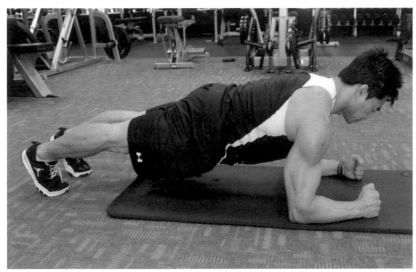

Core Exercise # 1: The Plank

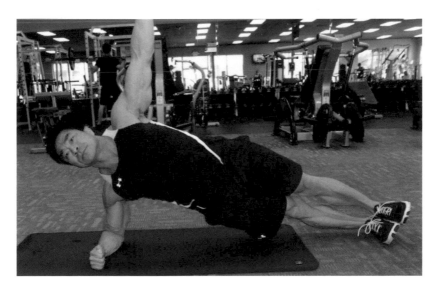

Core Exercise #2

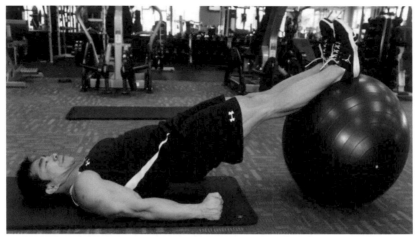

Core Exercise #3

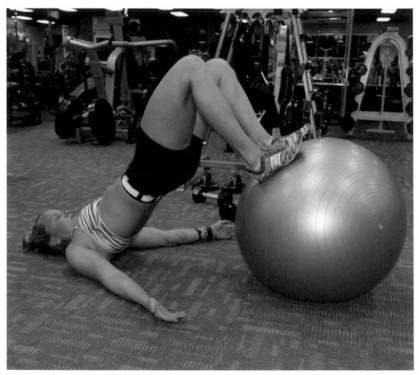

Core Exercise #4

Core muscle exercises should be started from static positions and then progressed to dynamic exercises.

Exercise Each Muscle in Your Body

The Centers for Disease Control (CDC) recommends that muscle-strengthening exercises for each major muscle group be done for two or more days per week. The major muscles can be easily divided into three simple groups: pushing, legs, and pulling. I recommend one day for each group, with a rest day in between. Muscles grow during the rest/recovery periods.

Monday: Pushing or chest, shoulders, triceps.

Tuesday: Rest and/or cardio.

Wednesday: Legs.

Thursday: Rest and/or cardio.

Friday: Pulling or back and biceps.

Saturday: Rest/cardio.

Sunday: Free—no exercise.

Begin each exercise day with five to 10 minutes of cardiovascular exercise as a warm up. Next, perform foam roller release followed by active/dynamic stretching. Then perform one or two core exercises.

The first exercise for each major muscle group is a warm up exercise, and is performed at 50%. Every fourth week, perform strength and stability exercises to strengthen the connective tissues. Stability exercises are performed while on an unstable surface, with the goal of activating stabilizers and trunk muscles.

Monday: Inclined 15 Degree Chest Press

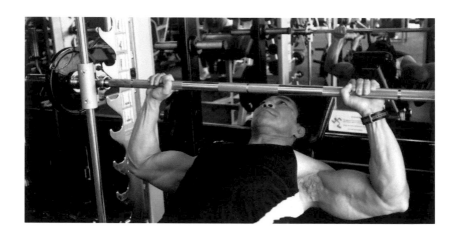

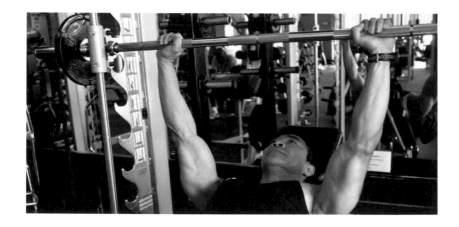

Monday: Seated Shoulder Press #1

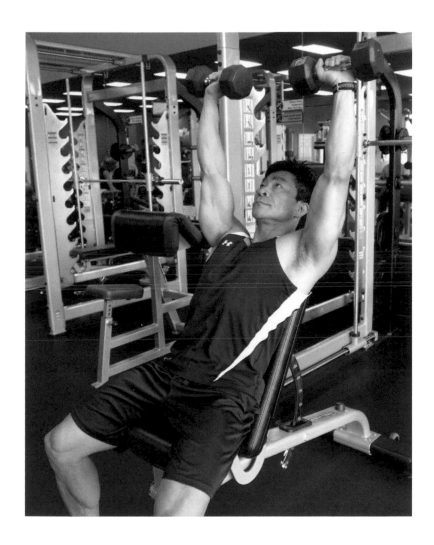

Monday: Seated Shoulder Press #2

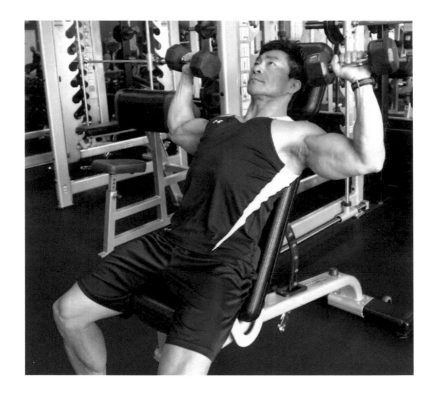

Monday: Triceps #1

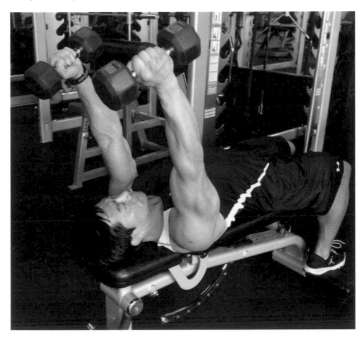

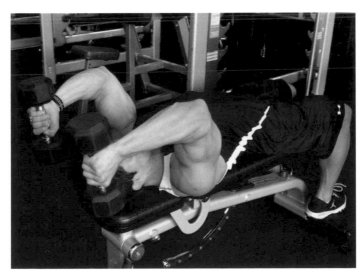

Wednesday: Leg Press #1

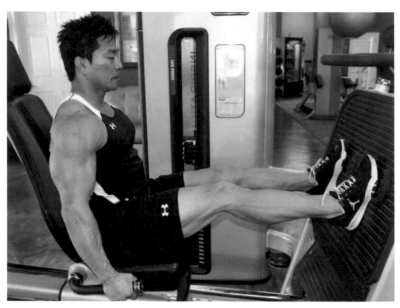

Wednesday: Leg Press #2

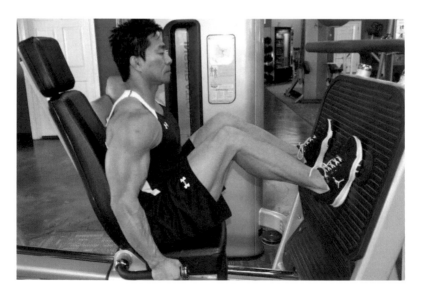

Wednesday: Legs—Smith Machine Squat

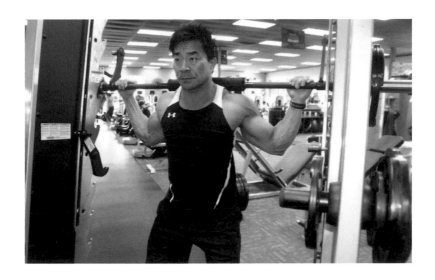

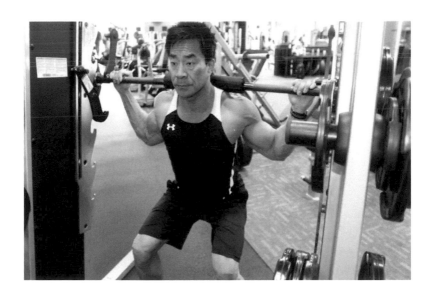

Wednesday: Leg Extensions

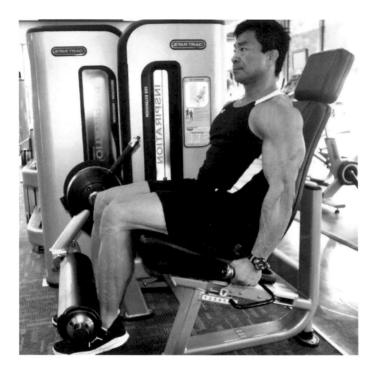

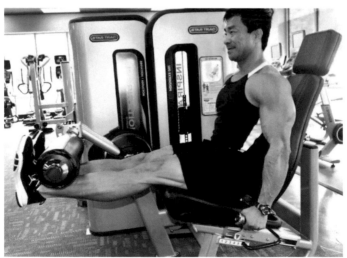

Wednesday: Legs—Hamstrings

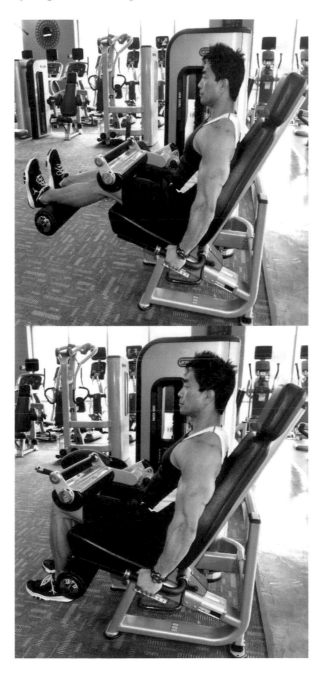

Friday: Back—Lat Pull-Down

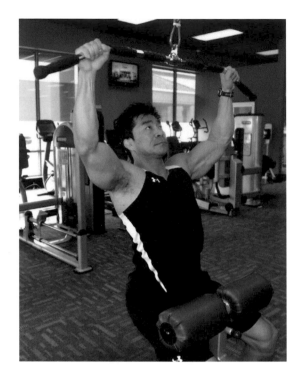

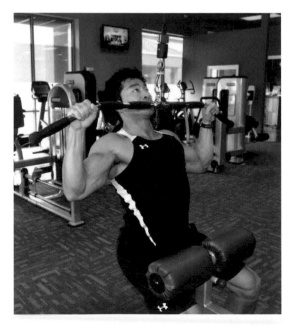

Friday: Back—Horizontal Row

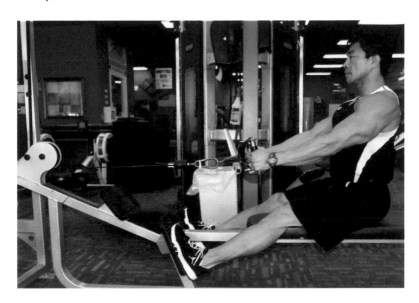

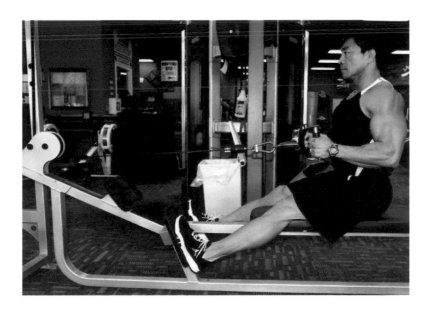

Friday: Biceps

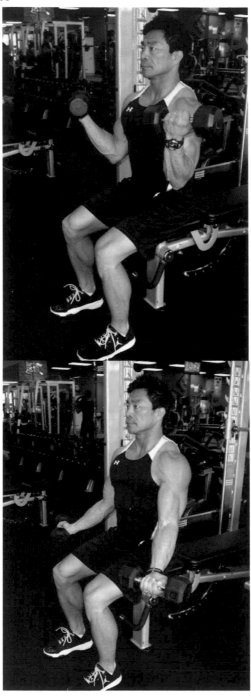

Monday & Friday: Abdominal Exercises

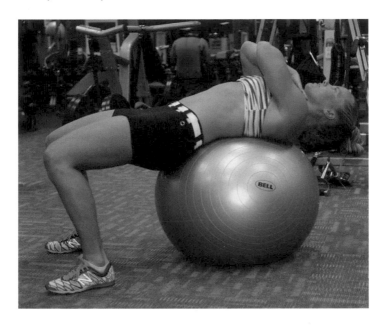

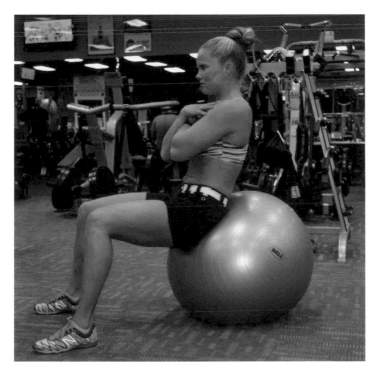

Monday & Friday: Abdominal Exercises

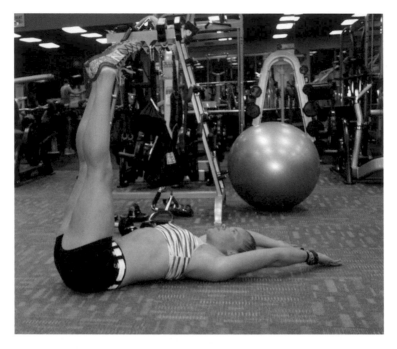

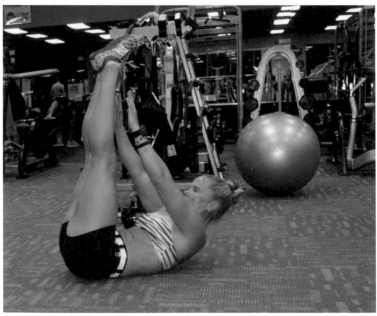

Abdominal muscles, like any other muscles, can be over-trained if exercised daily. These muscles need rest to grow; therefore, exercising two or three times a week is sufficient.

Core exercises that precede every workout also strengthen your abdominal muscles.

In order to visibly see your abdominal muscles ("six-pack abs") is more a question of your percentage of body fat than muscle bulk. You must be under 10% body fat in order to see your abdominal muscles. Thus, your diet is the key to having visible six-pack abs. Age and sex are not a factor—only body fat is; we all have abdominal muscles, but few of us are lean enough for them to be visible.

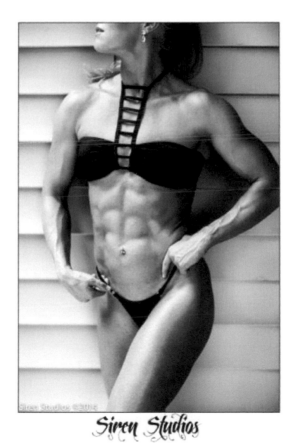

Six-Pack Abdominal Muscles With 8% Body Fat

It will take a minimum of three months of resistance training, training to muscle failure three to four sessions per week, to realize an increase in strength. (Kubo K, et al. (2010). *J Strength Cond Res*. 2:322-331.) It will take approximately six months to be able to visually observe changes.

You'll *feel* better within two weeks, because you're using more muscles, improving insulin sensitivity, and raising testosterone levels. Almost any physical activity will help to extend your life. Just 30 minutes of moderate activity four days a week, or twenty minutes of vigorous activity three times per week, will increase one's life span by 27% in both men and women aged 50 to 70 years. (Leitzmann MF, et al. (2007). *Arch Int Med*. 167(22):2453-2460.)

In addition to living longer, exercise helps to prevent disease. According to the American Heart Association, "Regular physical activity using large muscle groups, such as walking, running, or swimming, produces cardiovascular adaptations that increase exercise capacity, endurance, and skeletal muscle strength." (*Circulation* (2003) 107:3109-3116.) Habitual physical activity also prevents the development of coronary artery disease (CAD), and reduces symptoms in patients with established cardiovascular disease. There is also evidence that exercise reduces the risk of other chronic diseases, including type 2 insulin-resistant diabetes, osteoporosis, obesity, depression, and cancer of the breast and colon.

Now you know that exercise is necessary, and you know how much exercising to do. What specific types of exercising should you do?

What Type of Exercise—Resistance or Endurance, Weights or Cardio?

The answer is that you need both resistance training and endurance training.

If you'd like to run a marathon, then cardiovascular training is more important; however, you'll still need to do build strong leg muscles with some weight training. If, however, you want to compete in bodybuilding, then weight training for each muscle group is most important; however, you'll still need the benefits of endurance training—insulin sensitivity and cardiovascular health. Most people need both, and what predominates is a personal choice.

Weight or resistance exercise builds muscle mass and strength. Cardiovascular exercise increases the use of oxygen in cells and leads to increased exercise capacity. If you decide to train for a serious endurance event, such as a marathon, you'll lose both body fat and muscle. This is because intense endurance exercises block the production of the muscle building enzyme mTOR. (Nader GA (2006). *Med Sci Sports Exerc*. 38(11):1965-1970.)

In order to obtain the benefits of *both* resistance and cardiovascular exercise, you need to vary your routine, *and* avoid doing both on the same day.

Heavy Weights With Few Repetitions? Light Weights With Frequent Repetitions?

The answer to this depends on your goal. If you desire to maintain muscle tone, *any* exercise to muscle failure will be sufficient, as long as your diet is adequate.

In order to build or maintain muscle mass, you'll need adequate amino acids (protein), adequate carbohydrates to provide cellular energy, and adequate fats to ensure normal hormone levels.

If you're dieting and have a calorie deficit, then high resistance repetitions may cause muscle loss, because endurance training with caloric restriction has been shown to decrease the enzymes required for muscle building and repair (the mTOR pathway). (Stefan M, et al. (2010). *J Nutr*. 140(4):745-751.)

If you want to build muscle, you have to continuously overload your muscles with heavy weights and increase muscle protein synthesis, while providing all the nutrients and hormones your body needs, including adequate protein, carbohydrates and fat.

Can Exercise be Harmful?

Strenuous exercise can cause menstrual disorders in women. (Bullen BA, et al. (1985). *N Eng J Med*. 312:1349-1353.) In this study, 28 exercise-naïve women were asked to run four to 10 miles per day for two menstrual cycles, and to engage in 3.5 hours of exercise every day. Only four of the 28 subjects had a normal menstrual cycle during these intense exercises. Thus, it was found that intense exercise can disturb reproductive function in women.

Long-term training for, and competing in, extreme endurance events—such as marathons and ironman distance triathlons—can cause transient acute volume overload of the right heart (atria and ventricle), leading to damage of the heart muscle and the development of cardiac arrhythmias. (O'Keefe JH, et al. (2012). Mayo Clin Proc. 87(6):587-595.)

A common problem found in endurance athletes is lower-extremity stress fractures. (Kahanov L, et al. (2015). J Sports Med. 6:87-95.) A stress fracture occurs when muscles become fatigued and are unable to absorb additional force. In time, fatigued muscle transfers the overload to the bone, causing a tiny crack (stress fracture) in the bone. Stress fractures of the lower extremities are common injuries among individuals who participate in high load-bearing endurance activities, such as long-distance running. Stress fracture incidence in runners approaches 16% of all injuries.

Perhaps the most dangerous complication of excessive exercise and dehydration is rhabdomyolysis. Rhabdomyolysis is the rapid death of muscle cells and the subsequent release of a dangerous protein (myoglobin) into the bloodstream, which can cause kidney damage and elevation of serum potassium that can adversely, possibly even fatally, affect the heart.

Schiff, et al., studied 44 runners who completed a 99 km road race, and found that 25 of the runners demonstrated increased blood levels of myoglobin. Myoglobin was detected in the post-race urine samples of only six runners. Acute renal failure was not observed in any of these subjects.

In another study, 24 athletes who had competed in a triathlon showed a dramatic rise in serum myoglobin and reported muscle pain, but none required hospitalization. (Schiff HB, et al. (1978). *Q J Med, New series XLVII* (188):463-472.)

Knee injuries are very common. This is usually caused by weak muscles in the legs, weak core muscles, and misalignment of the knees in relation to the feet.

Shoulder muscles are also easily injured, because the shoulder joint is not designed for weight bearing and is made from the confluence of soft tissues. Preventing shoulder injuries requires strict adherence to form and technique. The muscles and tendons surrounding the shoulder joint keep the head of the upper arm bone firmly in the rotator cuff (the shallow socket of the shoulder). Any injury to these soft tissues can cause the upper arm bone to strike or impinge on the shoulder bone, causing pain.

Muscles weakened from years of disuse are easily injured. If pain occurs during a leg or shoulder exercise, it's best to immediately stop the exercise, rest and ice the muscle, apply a compression garment and, if possible, elevate the extremity. If pain persists, you may need to visit your physician.

Intense exercise requires a recovery period. Inadequate recovery and continued exercise stress leads to tissue damage.

Lower back injuries are common when first beginning an exercise routine. The core muscles connect the chest to the pelvis. Weak core muscles cannot maintain proper spinal alignment, resulting in lower back pain and injury. Back injuries can be prevented with proper warm up exercises and strong core muscles. When exercising, you should always schedule rest days in between weight-training days.

Treatment of most lower back pain includes rest, over-the-counter anti-inflammatory medications such as ibuprofen, massage therapy, acupuncture, and chiropractic treatments. Core muscle strength is the best protection against lower back injury.

If pain persists and prevents routine daily activity, then you need to see your doctor. Surgery is always the last resort.

How to Choose a Personal Trainer

If you can afford a personal trainer, do it. Even if your lessons are few and all you learn is how to use gym equipment, your body will benefit.

Finding a good trainer isn't easy. Your trainer must be certified by an established organization, such as the American Council on Exercise (ACE), National Academy of Sports Medicine (NASM), International Sports Science Association (ISSA), American College of Sports Medicine (ACSM), or National Strength and Conditioning Association (NSCA). It's ideal of your trainer has had additional post-certification training in human muscle kinetics.

You can tell a good trainer from a bad one by making a few simple observations. Your trainer should focus entirely upon you during your session, and not be conversing with other people. He or she should answer your questions with ease.

Your trainer should evaluate your abilities, ask you for your goals, and provide a road map so you can attain those goals. If your trainer doesn't guide you through dynamic stretching, you have the wrong trainer. A good trainer will integrate a corrective strategy into your program and help to prevent injuries while you pursue your fitness goals.

Your trainer should evaluate your current posture and joint movement—the musculoskeletal dysfunction that you're bringing into the gym from you current lifestyle. What you bring into the gym may cause injuries in the future, and these need to be prevented.

Two simple observations: your posture, both standing still when sitting, reveals important information. Your trainer should look for the three common patterns of dysfunction: flat feet and knock-knees; forward pelvic tilt; and rounded shoulders with head forward. (Clark M, et al., Editors (2014). *NASM Essentials of Personal Fitness Training*. Jones and Bartlett Learning 134-141.)

Posture, Standing Still: Flat Feet & Knock-Knees

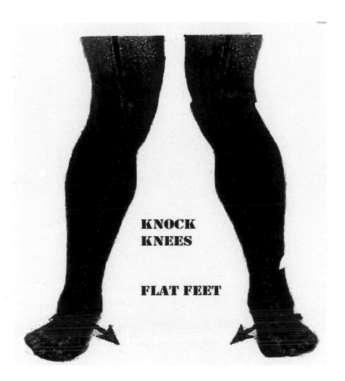

This dysfunction can lead to foot pain, shin splints, knee pain and lower back pain.

Forward Pelvic Tilt

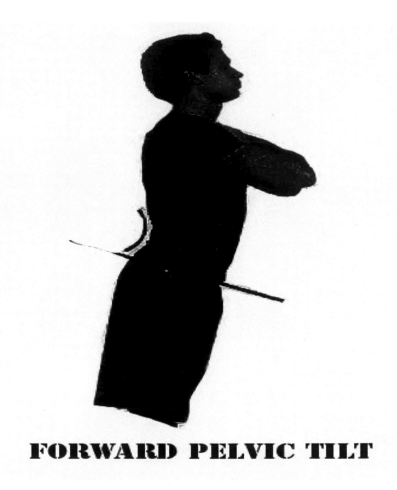

FORWARD PELVIC TILT

This dysfunction leads to hamstring (three posterior upper thigh muscles) injuries and pain, knee pain, and lower back pain.

Rounded Shoulders & Forward Head

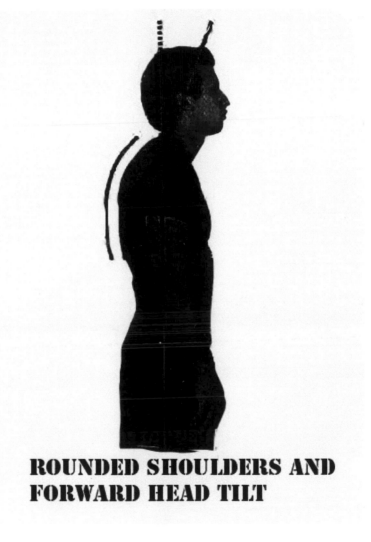

ROUNDED SHOULDERS AND
FORWARD HEAD TILT

This dysfunction leads to headaches, bicep tendonitis, shoulder (rotator cuff) pain, and numbness and pain in the neck, hands and fingers.

Your posture when sitting (dynamic posture) will provide additional information regarding muscle strength or weakness, balance, and joint movement.

Dynamic Posture Assessment

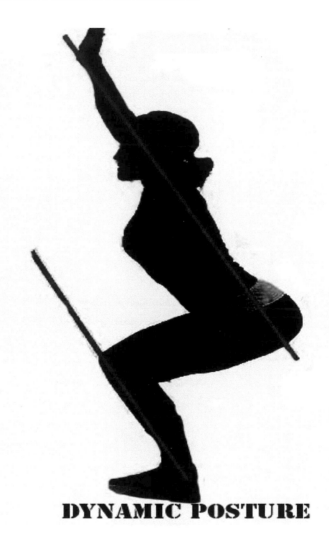

Dynamic and static posture evaluations will provide information which allows your trainer to select the appropriate training exercises to correct your specific weaknesses. There are many dynamic exercises available.

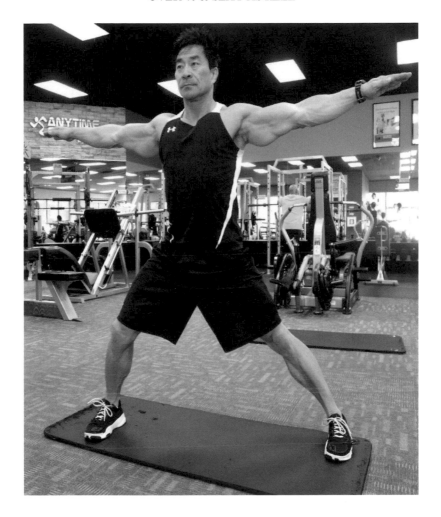

Donny H. Kim, Master Trainer, PES, CPT-NASM

CHAPTER 6

HOW TO LOSE FAT AND BUILD MUSCLE: DIET AS IT RELATES TO EXERCISE

The Holy Grail—How to Lose Fat and Build Muscle at the Same Time

With athletes who are involved in resistance training and dieting to lose body fat, the speed of weight loss is the important factor in the preservation of muscle mass. (Garthe et al. (2011 Apr). *Int J Sport Nutr Exerc Metab*. 21(2):97-104.)

Losing approximately one pound per week or precisely 0.7% of your body weight per week may be ideal. It's possible to increase lean body mass by 0.2% with this slow regimen of dieting and strength training.

Loss of approximately two pounds per week or 1.7% of your body weight per week causes no gain or slight loss of lean body mass.

The place to start your diet, as previously mentioned, is to first calculate how many calories per day you need in order to maintain your current weight. Then take this number and subtract 500 calories; this is your caloric starting point. This number will now be converted into proteins per day, carbohydrates per day, and fats per day.

The next calculation involves calories devoted to protein. The minimum protein intake for active athletes is 1.4 grams of protein intake for every 2.203 pounds of body weight. A diet higher in protein, such as 25% to 30% of total calories, will decrease appetite and increase satiety. In simple terms, you won't be hungry, and you'll eat less.

High-protein diets produce a sustained decrease in ad lib caloric intake that may be mediated by increased central nervous system leptin sensitivity, and results in significant weight loss. This anorexic effect of protein may contribute to the weight loss produced by low-carbohydrate diets. (Weigle DS, et al. (2005). *Am J Clin Nutr*. 82(1):41-48.) Dieting athletes require a relatively high protein intake to minimize loss of lean body mass.

As mentioned earlier, fat accompanies most protein sources, and the minimum fat content in your diet should be 15% of all calories. The remaining calories in your diet are for carbohydrates—40% to 60% of your total caloric intake per day. Carbohydrate minimum should be 3g/kg per day. (Burke LM, et al. *J Sports Science*. 29 (*sup.1*) 17-27.) Fat should not be lower than 15% to 20% of total caloric intake.

A "refeed" consists of a brief overfeeding period during which caloric intake is raised slightly above maintenance levels, wherein the increase in caloric intake is predominantly achieved by increasing carbohydrate consumption. Athletes such as bodybuilders and figure competitors may abandon their strict diets one day each week.

The proposed goal of this periodic refeeding is to temporarily increase circulating leptin and stimulate the metabolic rate. There is evidence indicating that leptin is acutely responsive to short-term overfeeding. (Chin-Chance C, et al. (2000). *J Clin Endocrinol Metab*. 85:2685-2691.)

Caffeine or coffee will help one lose body fat; see the section on supplements.

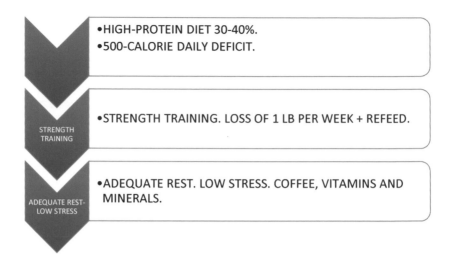

- •HIGH-PROTEIN DIET 30-40%.
- •500-CALORIE DAILY DEFICIT.

STRENGTH TRAINING

- •STRENGTH TRAINING. LOSS OF 1 LB PER WEEK + REFEED.

ADEQUATE REST-LOW STRESS

- •ADEQUATE REST. LOW STRESS. COFFEE, VITAMINS AND MINERALS.

Fat Loss—Muscle Gain—The Holy Grail

In order to build muscle tissue, your sex hormone levels and thyroid hormone levels must be in the normal range, preferably in the upper ranges of normal. This is essential.

Example of My Fat Loss Holy Grail Diet

My basal resting calories are approximately 1,800 calories per day, so 1,800 – 500 = 1,300 calories to lose <1 lb per day.

BREAKFAST: 5:00 a.m.—½ cup Quaker old-fashioned oatmeal made with water and ¼ apple, 1 protein shake, 1 tablespoon MCT (medium chain triglycerides) oil (such as coconut oil), and my supplements (multivitamins, 81 mg ASA (acetylsalicylic acid—low-dose aspirin), calcium with Vitamin D, creatine, HMB (beta-hydroxy beta-methylbutyric acid), CoQ10, and minerals) = 532 calories.

Total breakfast: 29 grams protein, 57 grams carbohydrates, 13.5 grams fat.

THE NEXT 3 MEALS: 6 ounces of chicken breast, ½ cup white rice, 200 grams of sweet potatoes, ad lib celery, radish, carrots and tomatoes = 528 calories.

DINNER: 6 ounces of chicken breast and salad = 200 calories.

Total calories = 1,285; total protein grams = 133 grams (41%); total carbohydrates = 132 grams (41%); total fat = 25 grams (17.5%).

Weight training as usual—each muscle group to complete failure— Monday pushing exercises; Wednesday legs; Friday pulling exercises. Cardiovascular exercises for 30 to 40 minutes each evening. If I wake up hungry between midnight and 3:00 a.m., I'll add a protein shake to help me return to sleep.

In summary, it's the result of <1 lb loss per week that you're looking for. This will give you an approximate starting place; you'll find that things change over time, and you'll need to adjust in order to succeed. Keep a written or digital (such as in your cell phone) journal every day, and keep the faith!

Carbohydrate Cycling—Extreme

Carbohydrate cycling is controversial and may not be needed by most athletes. There have been no prospective or randomized studies proving the benefit of carbohydrate cycling. If it works for you, then it's good.

The idea is similar to the concept of refeeding. You'll will lose body fat quickly on a low-carb diet; leptin decreases, your brain lowers the metabolic rate, and muscle synthesis decreases due to the lack of glycogen stores (low cellular energy).

Fat loss plateaus as your body seeks to remain constant (homeostasis). When you increase carbohydrate intake, leptin levels increase as fat cells are replenished and you'll be able to build muscle with a greater source of cellular energy from glycogen.

The purpose of cycling carbohydrates is to benefit from both fat loss and muscle gain by eating more carbohydrates on days of strenuous exercise and decreasing carbohydrates on days of rest or less strenuous exercise.

A typical carbohydrate cycle might look like this:

Day 1:   200 grams carbs (800 calories)—chest/pushing exercises

Day 2:   100 grams carbs (400 calories)—rest or 30 minutes cardio

Day 3:   200 grams carbs (800 calories)—leg exercises

Day 4:   100 grams carbs (400 calories)—rest or 30 minutes cardio

Day 5:   200 grams carbs (800 calories)—back/pulling exercises

Days 6&7: Variable, depending on results.

It's important to adjust your carbohydrate intake to meet your goals. A daily diary of your body measurements is helpful. Carbohydrate cycling may benefit most athletes trying to lose body fat, whose body fat is already below 10%—these are extreme bodybuilders.

The best sources of carbohydrates are oatmeal, grits, yams, potatoes, brown rice and cream of wheat. Fibrous carbohydrates, such as salads and most vegetables, can be eaten freely without measure. Avoid wheat products as discussed in another section—NO bread or pasta.

"I Joined a Gym, I Exercise, and I Look the Same"— Anthony's Story

Anthony is a 48-year-old owner of a software company. He's been going to the gym three days a week and lifting weights with his friends. He states that he has a healthy diet, and doesn't eat desserts or fried foods.

Anthony complains that his body image hasn't changed in two years—in fact, he's been gaining weight, and has been unable to lose his "love handles"(abdominal fat overhanging his pants), as well as being unable to see the six-pack abs that he had in high school.

When he was in high school he weighed 150 pounds, and now—30 years later—he weighs 185 pounds, with a BMI of 28.

His blood work showed normal kidney and liver function, normal free and total testosterone, normal estradiol, normal HGB-A1C, elevated triglycerides, slightly elevated LDL and slightly low HDL. His blood pressure was elevated, at 150/90.

His physical exam was normal, with no visible or palpable evidence of disease. A review of his family history indicated that his father developed coronary heart disease at age 66.

With a BMI above 25, Anthony is over-weight, not yet obese. He hasn't yet developed any measurable metabolic damage, but with hypertension, abnormal lipids and excess body fat, he's at risk for future arteriosclerosis, hypertension, coronary artery disease and stroke.

Like many, Anthony didn't calculate his caloric intake. Using a daily food diary, I calculated that he'd been consuming approximately 3,000 calories per day—a caloric excess of approximately 400 calories per day.

The exercises he'd been doing at the gym were high repetitions with light weights, and his gym days were more of a social meeting with friends than anything else. He did 60 minutes of light cardiovascular exercise on a treadmill before lifting weights. He actually only visited the gym twice a week, and rarely, if ever, exercised his legs; and he *never* exercised his core muscles.

Anthony was making many mistakes.

1. He was consuming too many calories, and so his body was making and storing body fat. In order to lose body fat, he requires a maximum of 2,100 calories per day (a 500 calorie deficit against his caloric maintenance level). He should aim to lose one pound per week.

2. His cardiovascular exercise was inefficient, since it didn't incorporate high-intensity interval training (HIIT).

3. Doing cardiovascular exercise *before* resistance or weight training shuts down the metabolic pathways to building muscle.

4. Weight training to build muscle must include heavy weights to continuously and progressively stress the muscle. More muscle increases metabolic rate and energy output.

5. Your legs have the biggest muscles in your body and provide a strong base, along with the core muscles, which allows you to increase upper-body muscle strength by using heavier weights. If your core and leg muscles are weak, you can't lift heavier weights; this limits your ability to build new muscle.

Anthony encountered much difficulty in changing his diet and lifestyle; we continue to struggle with his identified problems.

CHAPTER 7
WHAT IS A DIETARY SUPPLEMENT?

Dietary supplements provide substances that may be needed but are missing from your diet. Supplements are not intended to treat disease; they're intended to ensure peak performance by adding something that may be missing from the foods you're eating. The most widely used supplements in the U.S. are multivitamins. (Madison Park; *"Half of Americans Use Supplements"* (10/3/15) CNN.)

One reason you may need supplements is that with vigorous exercise, your body needs time to recover, repair itself and build new muscle. Supplements may help your body to recover and prevent injuries.

Most supplements are not needed if you don't regularly do vigorous exercise, since a *balanced diet* can provide all essential nutrients. If you're eating a high-protein diet and are exercising vigorously, you shouldn't consider yourself to be part of the general population; scientific population studies of supplements don't apply to you! You're an athlete, and an exception to the rule.

Many recommendations for supplements may be logical from a

theoretical perspective, but lack human prospective studies. Thus, many supplements are without a robust scientific basis.

According to Professor Marina Heinon of the University of Helsinki, 90% of health claims made by dietary supplements are incorrect. (*Ravintolisissa paljon humpuukia*. Yle.fi (2012) 1710.)

FDA Regulations

In the U.S., the Food and Drug Administration (FDA) overseas the safety of food, drugs and cosmetics. The rules they have promulgated regarding drugs that are intended to treat disease are far different than the rules regarding dietary food supplements. Today, the FDA usually requires a new drug to show superiority to the current standard of care, using human prospective randomized studies. For a new drug to show 10% superiority usually requires a minimum of 400 patients.

According to *Forbes* magazine, the average cost of developing a new drug is at least $4 billion. (Matthew Herper; *Forbes/Business*; 2/10/12.)

The costs of developing and bringing food supplements to market are minimal. No government approval is needed to make and sell a dietary food supplement, so caveat emptor—buyer beware. Canadian investigators using DNA barcoding tested 44 bottles of popular supplements sold by 12 companies. They found that 33% were not what they claimed to be. (O'Connor A (11/3/13). *The New York Times*.)

Levels of Scientific Evidence

Level I—Prospective randomized trials agree—the most reliable information.

Level II—At least one prospective randomized trial is positive, but possibly imperfect design; disagreement in controlled studies—reliable information.

Level III—Case studies, retrospective data, historical data; possibly helpful information.

Level IV—Case studies, limited numbers, controversial information.

Level V—Expert opinion, controversial information.

In my medical practice, I'm required to use Level I or II evidence-based treatments for my sick patients. If this information is not available, then I use Level III or IV information; however, insurance companies frequently won't cover therapy based on Level III or higher data. What is written on a medication's package insert, and what insurance companies will pay for, is always Level I or II evidence.

Listed below are mostly over-the-counter supplements that you can purchase in vitamin shops and grocery stores. There are a few prescription drugs also included in this list, as well.

Whey Protein (Level I)—Yes

Whey protein and casein are the proteins found in cow's milk. When renin is added to milk, the casein and whey separate, leaving the whey protein in solution and the casein solidifying into cheese. Both products are used in making protein supplements.

Whey protein is rapidly absorbed. Whey protein supplementation before and after resistance training sessions provide significantly greater improvement in exercise recovery both 24 and 48 hours post-exercise than found in subjects ingesting a placebo. (Hoffman J, et al. (2008). *JISSN*. 5(1):6.)

There are multiple studies showing that whey protein rapidly stimulates protein synthesis and increases muscle hypertrophy. Whey protein is best taken early post-exercise. (Phillips SM (June 2010). *Summer Meeting Nutrition Society*, Edinburgh.) This is not controversial—whey protein after exercise *will* help you build muscle.

According to the EFSA Panel on Dietetic Products, Nutrition and Allergies (*EFSA Journal* (2010) 8(10):1818), a cause-and-effect relationship has not been established between the consumption of whey protein and growth or maintenance of muscle mass over and above the well-established role of protein on the claimed effect. This complex language simply states that *any* source of protein will do. However, there's more to protein supplements and foods than just amino acids. You need to be careful which protein powder you choose—some of the popular protein products may contain relatively high amounts of cadmium, arsenic, lead and mercury, and these are not listed on the package. (See Consumer Reports (October, 2010).)

I recommend whey powders from farms in New Zealand, since these cows are grass-fed and given no antibiotics. Cows that are fed high-grain diets have a higher incidence of metabolic disorders related to the build up of several toxic and inflammatory compounds, as well as changes in amino acid profiles in their digestive fluids, as compared to cows on low-grain diets. Having these metabolic complications (and the subsequent need for antibiotics) negatively affects the quality of dairy products produced, including the whey protein found in milk. (Saleem, et al. (2012). *J Dairy Sci.* 98(1).)

Why do farmers in the U.S. feed their cows grain? Farmers have turned to grains—such as corn—due to convenience and money. They confine cows to feedlots, feed them grains, and also feed them antibiotics and the enzymes necessary to digest grains, since cows are normally unable to digest grains! The cows rapidly gain weight and yield a higher return on investment (more money). The quality of the milk may suffer.

Fish Oil (Level II)—Yes

Fish oil contains two essential omega 3 fatty acids that our bodies need and must obtain from food: docosahexaenoic acid (DHA), and eicosapentaenoic acid (EPA). These essential fatty acids are present in salmon, mackerel, sardines, flaxseeds, chia seeds, walnuts and canola oil. You need them.

Populations with high intakes of omega 3 (n 3) polyunsaturated fatty acids (such as the Inuit) have low rates of heart disease. This observation has increased the interest in the possible benefit of fish oils. (Harper CR, Jacobson TA. *Arch Intern Med.* 161(18):2185.) Fish oil concentrate administered at high doses can reduce levels of triglycerides in patients with HIV and hypertriglyceridemia. (Harris WS, Connor WE, Illingworth DR, et al. (1990). *Effects of fish oil on VLDL triglyceride kinetics in humans. J Lipid Res.* 31:1549.)

Other types of omega 3 supplements, such as flax seeds, have not been adequately studied.

Negative fish oil data comes from a study that evaluated prostate cancer prevention in men taking selenium and Vitamin E. (Brasky TM, et al. (2013). *JNCI*. 10.) The study was negative, but did reveal an increased prostate cancer risk in men with higher blood levels of long chain polyunsaturated fatty acids. This was based on a single blood test, and was neither randomized nor prospective (Level III or IV).

Furthermore, taking fish oil supplements did not improve the natural history of patients with known coronary risk factors. (Roncaglioni MC, et al. (May 9, 2013). *NEJM*.)

There are multiple studies that do show that a combination of fish oil and exercise increases protein synthesis in muscle cells, and improves insulin sensitivity. (Heikkinen A, et al. (2009). *Int J Sport Nutr Diet*. 100:1-21; Sanchez-Benito JL, et al. (2007). Nutr Hosp. 22(5):552-559.)

Fish oil has anabolic properties and is useful in building muscle, despite not being able to improve heart disease and possibly increasing prostate cancer risk. The choice is yours. I take fish oil.

Creatine (Level II)—Yes, With Caution

Creatine makes more ATP in the mitochondria available for muscular activity, and this longer duration of muscle contraction enhances the power of athletes over a short period of time.

Creatine is not important for endurance athletes.

Taking approximately 20 grams of creatine per day over a seven-day period shows a measurable increase in power production during short-duration resistance exercises to muscle failure.

Creatine has not been shown to improve long-duration endurance exercise. Elevated muscle creatine enhances exercise performance by matching ATP supply to ATP demand.

An increase in body weight from one to two pounds is common after one week of creatine supplementation, due to an increase in intracellular water.

There is little data on long-term creatine use. Creatine allows users to train more intensely. Few adverse side effects have been found with creatine use in healthy individuals. (Kraemer WL, Volek JS (July 1, 1999). *Sports Medicine Clinics*, Elsevier.)

Furthermore, a meta-analysis performed at the University of Regina, Saskatchewan, Canada, in 2014 showed that the addition of creatine supplementation realized an improvement in both bone mineral density and muscle growth in older adults doing resistance training.

If you have a history of renal dysfunction, you should not take creatine, as it will increase the serum creatinine that your physician uses to measure your renal function.

I recommend the minimum maintenance dose of 1 2 grams per day, along with frequent vacations from use, for older adults.

DHEA (Level III)—Still a Question; Possibly Yes

Dehydroepiandrosterone (DHEA) is a commercially available supplement aimed at improving libido and wellbeing. There is little evidence to support the use of DHEA for this purpose. DHEA is a precursor element for the production of androgens and estrogens in non-reproductive tissues.

Levels of DHEA decline with age. It has been postulated that restoring the circulating levels of DHEA to those that are found in young people may have anti-aging effects and improve wellbeing and sexual function. There is no randomized prospective scientific data to support this.

There is some positive data in patients with adrenal insufficiency. Studies of DHEA therapy in patients with adrenal insufficiency suggest that this group is the most likely to derive health benefits from DHEA supplementation.

There is one interesting positive study. (Yen, et al. (1995). *Annals of the New York Academy of Sciences*. 774:128-142.) In this study, men and women over the age of 50 took 50 mg of DHEA daily. DHEA levels rose to those of young adults within two weeks.

The subjects then had their immune systems assessed through the measurement of lymphocytes, T cells, and natural killer cells. The DHEA increased the levels of these cells by 67% in men and 84% in women.

A follow up study using 100 mg of DHEA showed that the subjects also experienced gains in lean body mass, as well as an increase in muscular strength. Male subjects also experienced a significant decrease in body fat.

There are no long-term studies of elderly subjects taking 100 mg of DHEA daily. I take this supplement; caveat emptor.

Testosterone (Level I)—Yes, But Only With an Expert; Controlled Substance

According to the U.S. Library of Medicine and the U.S. Institute of Health, testosterone is a hormone made by the testicles in men. It's the most important androgen (male) hormone in the body. Women produce a smaller amount, converting estrogen to testosterone by way of the enzyme aromatase. Testosterone is essential for both men and women. Androgens, such as testosterone, are often referred to as steroids or anabolic steroids.

Testosterone is important for both men and women:

- Keeping bones and muscles strong;

- Making sperm;

- Maintaining sex drive;

- Making red blood cells; and

- Feeling well, and having energy in general.

As you become older, testosterone levels slowly drop. This can lead to various symptoms, including:

- Low sex drive;

- Problems having an erection;

- Low sperm count;

- Sleep problems, such as insomnia;

- Decrease in muscle size, strength and bone density;

- Increase in body fat;

- Depression; and

- Trouble concentrating.

Who Should Try Testosterone Therapy?

To help assess whether testosterone therapy is right for you, your doctor will likely do the following:

- Measure your testosterone levels one or more times.

- Make sure there are no other causes of your symptoms. These include side effects from medicines, thyroid problems, depression, or overuse of alcohol.

If your testosterone level is low, your doctor will discuss the risks and benefits of testosterone therapy and how this therapy may help you.

In my opinion, most physicians are not knowledgeable regarding testosterone, and are hesitant to prescribe testosterone, which is a controlled substance. They will tell you that the signs and symptoms of low testosterone are part of the "normal aging process."

If you wish to age "normally," you're reading the wrong book. In men and women over 40 years of age, maintaining sufficient levels of testosterone in the blood is an important part of building muscle, increasing activity level, losing body fat, and increasing endurance. Your blood levels should be checked by an expert: total testosterone, free testosterone, estradiol, IGF 1, TSH, lipid profile with LDL subsets, PSA, CBC, and CMP.

If your testosterone levels are low, the best replacement is by way of a testosterone cypionate injection, since this is long-acting (four to six days) and is similar to the testosterone made by your body. It does not require liver activation, as do testosterone pills and creams, and so does not add stress to your liver.

Testosterone and estradiol levels must be monitored frequently, because some of the added testosterone will be aromatized to estrogen.

Testosterone is a hormone and a ligand (a molecule that binds to another, usually larger, molecule). Like any other ligand, in chronic excess, cells may become immune to its actions and cause pathology. There are no scientific data linking testosterone to either prostate or breast cancer. However, testosterone accelerates the growth of prostate cancer, should it already be present. Among a group of men in the Veterans Administration healthcare system who underwent coronary angiography and had a low serum testosterone level, the use of testosterone therapy was associated with an increased risk of adverse outcomes. (Vigan R, et al. (2013). *JAMA*. 310(17):1829-1836.) This VA study demonstrated a 5.8% increased risk of cardiovascular events over a period of three years—Level II data.

Thus, despite the improvement in sexual function, bone mineral density, decreased body fat, increased strength, improved lipid profiles and decreased insulin resistance, there is an increased incidence of mortality with testosterone supplementation. This study did not evaluate type of testosterone supplements, estradiol levels or free testosterone blood levels. This 5.8% increase in this study of men can likely be attributed to elevated estradiol levels, a known cardiac risk factor.

Caveat emptor.

Human Chorionic Gonadotropin (hCG) (Level IV)—No for Weight Loss, No for Fat Loss

hCG is indicated in men to prevent testicular atrophy associated with the long-term use of testosterone. Under normal conditions, the testicles produce testosterone. If testosterone levels drop and are supplemented with exogenous testosterone in order to maintain normal blood levels, the brain detects the change and stops stimulating the testicles (by way of luteinizing hormone, LH) to produce testosterone.

In this setting, the testicles may atrophy from disuse. The addition of hCG stimulates the testicles to continue producing testosterone (hCG mimics LH), and thus prevents atrophy. In males, hCG alone, without testosterone supplementation, can increase the production of testosterone by the testicles. Thus, hCG can be used alone to restore normal levels. hCG is not a controlled substance; however, the need for medical experts is essential if you wish to increase testosterone.

The use of hCG in women is more complicated, and since women do not have testicles, hCG will not increase testosterone production. In both women and men, the controversy is really regarding weight loss and the "hCG diet."

Since the hCG diet contains 500 to 1,000 calories per day, all of the benefits achieved on the hCG diet can be attributed to caloric restriction. A review study refuting the hCG diet has been published in the *American Journal of Clinical Nutrition*, concluding that hCG is neither safe nor effective as a weight-loss aid. (Stein MR, et al. *Am J Clin Nutr.* 29(9):940-948.) hCG will not selectively increase fat loss or preserve muscle mass during weight reduction.

Beta-Hydroxy Beta-Methylbutyrate (HMB) (Level III)—Yes

HMB (B hydroxyl B methylbutyrate) is an effective supplement for adults to increase lean body mass, according to a meta-analysis and multiple scientific studies. (Vukovich MD, et al. (2001). J Nutr. 131:2049-2052.) HMB and a mixture of other branch chain amino acids improve protein metabolism and increase lean body mass in elderly and chronically ill subjects.

HMB benefits people who exercise vigorously (defined as three weeks or more of resistance training two or more times a week). (Nissen SL, Sharp RL (2003). *J App Physiology.* 94(2):651-659.)

HMB has data supporting its use to augment lean mass and strength gains with resistance training. The benefits of this supplement have been confirmed by meta-analysis.

Vitamin D and Calcium (Level II)—Yes

According to the National Institutes of Health, Office of Dietary Supplements, older adults are at increased risk of developing Vitamin D insufficiency. Older skin cannot synthesize Vitamin D efficiently. Many adults spend little time outdoors, and they may have inadequate dietary intake of this vitamin.

Your body is designed to manufacture Vitamin D when sunlight shines on your skin. In the presence of a low Vitamin D level, your body may lose bone density and you could be at risk for bone fractures.

The loss of height in many older adults is due to loss of bone density and the decrease in size of the bones in the spine. Exercise is also important in maintaining bone density in the weight-bearing bones of your body. Many adults in the U.S. who experience hip fractures have low serum Vitamin D levels (<30 nmol/L; <12 ng/mL).

Osteoporosis is a pathological loss of bone density (2.5 standard deviations from a healthy bone, as measured on a "DEXA" scan), requiring medical treatment to prevent fractures. Osteopenia is much more common condition (there is less bone loss than with osteoporosis), and can be treated with non-prescription calcium and Vitamin D supplements, along with weight-bearing exercises. Weight-bearing exercises include walking, running, lifting and dancing. Swimming does not strengthen your bones.

Medium Chain Triglycerides (MCT) (Level III)—Yes for Body Fat Loss

Medium chain triglycerides (MCT) are made from coconut and palm kernel oils. They differ from the saturated fats found in meat and dairy, owing to their ability to rapidly enter the blood circulation and go directly to the liver.

Normal fats must be digested slowly, requiring chylomicrons (lipoprotein particles that transport dietary lipids from the intestines to other locations in the body) and slow lymphatic transport. MCT are rapidly metabolized into an energy source, and less fat from this source is stored in fat cells—so less fat accumulates. (St. Onge M P, Jones PJ (2002). *J Nutr.* 132(3):329-332.)

MCT cause significant weight loss, lower fat deposition, and decreased appetite due to increased satiety. More research needs to be done regarding the long-term benefits of MCT.

Resveratrol (Level V)—Too Early to be Certain; Caveat Emptor

Resveratrol has become famous as the ingredient in red wine that will makes you live longer. (Smoliga JM, et al. (2011). *Molecular Nutrition and Food Research.* 55(8):1129-1141.) Many claim that resveratrol will also prevent the metabolic diseases of aging and prevent cancer by gene activation.

Many studies have shown that resveratrol has anti-aging, anti-carcinogenic, and anti-inflammatory effects in laboratory animals. This might be relevant to humans, but human data is not yet available. The limited human clinical trials to date only attest to resveratrol's safety and bioavailability.

Soy (Level III)—Useful Protein Source for Some, Not All

Soy is a useful source of protein for some, but not all, and much research continues. (Barrett JR (2006 June). *Environ Health Perspect.* 114(6):352-358.)

Soy products are frequently found in grocery stores throughout the U.S. and are mostly consumed by infants, vegetarians and Asians. In Korea, Japan, China and Indonesia, soy proteins are more popular. Soy protein, unlike other vegetable proteins, contains all the essential amino acids and is thus is an important food.

Soy contains isoflavones, which are plant estrogens, and these have numerous effects on the human body that are not found in animal protein sources. Soy isoflavones are controversial and are currently being researched, since estrogens can alter cell function, including cell cycle, fertility and ovarian function, in animal studies.

In humans, soy products are commonly found in baby foods, and no negative effects have yet to be found in adults who were fed soy baby foods when they were young.

With regard to the cardiovascular benefits of soy proteins, there is a minor reduction in low-density lipoproteins (LDL).

The real potential danger of isoflavones occurs in breast tissue, where breast secretions and cell proliferation are increased—a potential sign of an increased risk of breast cancer.

In summary, soy products are good sources of protein and good sources of fiber for most people.

Statins and Red Rice Yeast (Level I)—These Prevent Heart Attacks in Patients With Coronary Artery Disease

Red rice yeast is an ancient Chinese and Japanese food and traditional medicine. It is obtained by cultivating fermented rice with a mold called Monascus purpureus. This traditional remedy was used to invigorate the body.

In a 2006 Chinese prospective randomized study of 5,000 patients with coronary artery disease, a Chinese standardized red rice yeast product reduced the incidence of repeat heart attacks by 45%, and reduced cardiac deaths by 31%.

The drug lovastatin (Mevacor), approved by the U.S. FDA to lower cholesterol and prevent heart attacks in patients with coronary artery disease, contains the identical compounds—monacolins—that are present in red rice yeast.

The current 2014 guidelines of the American College of Cardiology recommends statins for anyone with existing coronary artery disease, an LDL OF 190 mg/dl or higher, type 2 diabetes in those aged 40 to 70 years, and anyone in the 40 to 70 year-old group with a 10 year, 7.5% risk of developing coronary artery disease. This last group of 7.5% risk is controversial and is Level IV evidence.

Coenzyme Q10 (CoQ10) (Level V)—Yes

Coenzyme Q10 is present in the mitochondria of every living cell in your body. The greater the metabolic activity of the cell, the greater the concentration of CoQ10.

According to the Mayo Clinic (mayoclinic.org), deficiencies of CoQ10 may cause heart failure and high blood pressure. There is good scientific evidence that treating these deficiencies with CoQ10 supplements is effective in improving chronic congestive heart failure and hypertension.

CoQ10 is a dietary supplement and thus not under federal regulation, and since it's available over-the-counter, it's unlikely that any prospective randomized studies will be done. In general, randomized studies are expensive to do and are done only when a drug can be patented and thus enable pharmaceutical companies to have a return on their investment.

It's very interesting to note that CoQ10 levels decrease with the use of cholesterol-lowering drugs (statins). This is a good reason to use statins or any cholesterol-lowering supplements *only* where Level I and Level II data exist, as in the case of men with coronary artery disease and/or diabetes.

Coffee (Level III)—Yes

Despite what critics say, caffeine can be healthy. Early studies showing coffee as harmful were done when the harmful effects of smoking were not taken into consideration; most coffee drinkers at that time also smoked cigarettes.

According to the Mayo Clinic, coffee may protect you from Parkinson's disease, diabetes and liver cancer. Coffee improves cognitive function and memory, and decreases the risk of depression by blocking the inhibitory neurotransmitter adenosine. (Fredholm BB (1995). *Pharmacology and Toxicology*. 76(2):93-101.)

Caffeine is a "fat burner," and can increase adrenaline levels and release fatty acids from the fat tissues. Coffee can increase your metabolic rate by 3 to 11%. (Dilloo AG, et al. (1989). *Am J Clin Nutr.* 49(10):44-50.) A cup of coffee can improve your performance in the gym by 11 to 12%. (Doherty M, Smith PM (2004). *Int J Sport Nutr Exerc Metab.* 6:626-646.)

Estrogen Replacement (Level II)—It Depends

The use of estrogen supplements during menopause is not ideal for every woman, but can be very helpful for some.

The benefits of estrogen replacement include relief of hot flashes, increase in bone density in refractory bone loss, increase in health, and longevity in early menopause (before age 40).

Estrogen replacement, however, *does* increase the incidence of breast cancer. (Hou N, et al. (2013). *J Natl Cancer Inst.* 105(18):1365-1372.) It's especially dangerous in women with a strong family history of breast cancer, as well as in women with dense breast tissue. Mammography may not visualize dense breast tissue well, and malignancies can be missed.

Probiotics (Level II)

Today there is much discussion of probiotics, and little prospective randomized data. Probiotics are living, nonpathogenic bacteria or yeast ingested to benefit the gastrointestinal tract and/or vagina.

Probiotics are not regulated by the FDA or any other governmental agency, and are available over-the-counter. Due to this liberal policy, there is little drug company interest in performing expensive randomized studies.

The most consistent data involves various strains of Lactobacillus. (Reid G (1999). *Appl Environ Microbiol.* 65(9):3763-3766.) *Lactobacillus rhamnosus GG* can reduce diarrhea. *L-NCFM* can improve lactose intolerance. *L. casei Shirota* and *L. MM53* decrease gastroenteritis caused by rotavirus. *L. GR 1* and *L. B 54* can restore vaginal microflora and prevent urinary tract infections. Some strains help to maintain remission status in inflammatory bowel disease.

Randomized studies have been done with *S. boulardii, L. rhamnosus,* and labs showed improvement in diarrhea caused by antibiotics. (Verna EC (2010). *Therap Adv Gastroenterol*. 3(5):307-319.)

Katherine's Story

Katherine is a 55-year-old married female. She has a full-time job with a marketing company and works five days a week. I saw her in follow-up for her breast cancer, and she had multiple new symptom complaints: headaches, fuzzy thinking, pains in her legs, and fatigue. In view of these new symptoms, I was compelled to evaluate her with blood tests and scans for recurrent breast cancer.

All of Katherine's tests were normal, yet her symptoms continued. Additional history revealed that her serum cholesterol was elevated at 250 mg/dl, and her primary care medical provider had placed her on Crestor (a statin), despite the fact that she had no family history of heart disease nor any personal history of chest pain or heart disease. She was not diabetic. Her lipid profile in my office indicated normal HDL and LDL.

I immediately discontinued her Crestor, and within four weeks, all of her symptoms disappeared.

The lesson here is that total cholesterol alone should never be used as the deciding factor in prescribing a statin.

CHAPTER 8
OVER-THE-COUNTER "FAT BURNERS"

The best thing about "fat burner" supplements is their names.

The "fat burner" concept is that there are substances which increase the use of fat as a source of energy for cells, causing one to lose body fat.

There are many supplements sold in stores called "fat burners" for which there is little or no scientific information. These include L carnitine, DHEA, yohimbe, garcinia cambogia and raspberry ketones.

Caffeine (Level I)—A True Fat Burner

In one controlled study, caffeine was found to have enhanced the endurance of long-distance bicyclists. This was due to the combined effects of caffeine on lipolysis (the breakdown of fats by hydrolysis to release fatty acids) and its positive influence on nerve impulse transmission.

In the bicyclists who had caffeine, there was a greater rate of lipid metabolism compared to the decaffeinated treatment group. Calculations of carbohydrate (CHO) metabolism from respiratory exchange data revealed that the subjects oxidized roughly 240 grams of CHO in both trials. Fat oxidation was significantly higher ($P < 0.05$) during the caffeine group than in the decaffeinated group. On average, the participants' rated their effort (perceived exertion scale) during the caffeine trial to be significantly easier ($P < 0.05$) than the demands of the decaffeinated group. (Costil DL, et al. (1978). *Med Sci Sports*. 10(3):155-158.)

Caffeine works by increasing the rate of fatty acid metabolism. If you drink coffee before you exercise, you'll use more calories from fat; thus, you will truly burn fat.

Ephedrine (Level II)—A Fat Burner

Ephedrine is a stimulant (sympathomimetic amine) that increases dopamine and noradrenaline in the brain. (Munhall AC, Johnson SW (2006). *Brain Res*. 1069(1):96-103.) Ephedrine promotes short-term weight loss. (Shekelle PG, et al. (2003). *JAMA*. 289(12):1537-1545.) Ephedrine is an FDA-controlled substance and is limited to the treatment of diseases such as asthma, bronchitis and allergies.

Caffeine and ephedrine are synergistic in weight-loss effect. (Magkos F, Kavouras SA (2004). *Sports Med NZ*. 34(13):871-889.) Ephedrine, caffeine and aspirin taken together are a popular combination used by bodybuilders to cut down on body fat before a competition.

Green Tea Extract (Level II)—Fat Burner

Green tea promotes fat oxidation beyond that attributable to its caffeine content . Green tea extract contains catechins (a type of disease-fighting flavonoid and antioxidant) that play a role in the control of body composition via sympathetic activation of thermogenesis, fat oxidation, or both. (Dulloo AG, et al. (1999). *Am J Clin Nutr*. 70(6):1040-1045.)

CHAPTER 9

THE MEDICAL MANAGEMENT OF OBESITY FROM THE DOCTOR'S POINT OF VIEW—LEVEL II DATA

The National Health and Nutrition Survey results (NHANES, 1999) estimate that 61% of U.S. adults are either overweight or obese; adult obesity nearly doubled during the 14 years of the study, increasing to 27%. (NHANES (1999). *U.S. National Center for Health Statistics, Prevalence of overweight and obesity among adults*. Hyattsville, MD: U.S. Department of Health and Human Services, Public Health Service, Centers for Disease Control and Prevention.)

Obesity is an independent risk factor for early mortality. Overall mortality begins to increase with BMI levels greater than 25, and increases most dramatically as BMI levels surpass 30. (Manson JE, Willett WC, Stampfer MJ, et al. (1995). *N Engl J Med*. 333:677-685.) The longer the duration of obesity, the higher the risk. (*Obesity: preventing and managing the global epidemic*. Report of a WHO consultation (2000). *World Health Organ Tech Rep Ser*. 894:i xii:1 253.)

Obesity predisposes a person to coronary artery disease by increasing blood pressure (hypertension), producing abnormal lipids, and increasing insulin resistance. In addition to heart disease, obesity causes sleep apnea and degenerative joint disease.

A modest weight loss of 10% of your body weight will reduce insulin resistance, lower blood pressure, and decrease abnormal lipid production. (Reisin E, Abel R, Modan M, Silverberg DS, Eliahou HE, Modan B (1978). *N Engl J Med*. 298:1 6; Wood PD, Stefanick ML, Dreon DM, et al. *N Engl J Med*. 319:1173 9.)

This book recommends diet and exercise together as the best treatment for obesity. In addition to diet and exercise, other treatments can include pharmacotherapy, behavior therapy and surgery. The surgical approach is discussed in another section.

A low-calorie diet of 500 to 1,000 calories below your maintenance calorie level will reduce total body weight by 8% over three to 12 months. A very low-calorie diet totaling 800 calories per day will produce very rapid weight loss, but cannot be maintained in the long term and after one year, is not superior to the above low-calorie approach. (*Clinical Guidelines on the Identification, Evaluation, and Treatment of Overweight and Obesity in Adults—The Evidence Report. National Institutes of Health* (published erratum appears in Obes Res. (1998) 6:464), *Obes Res*. (1998) 6 Suppl 2:51S-209S.)

Exercise at 60% to 85% of estimated maximum heart rate over three to seven 30 to 60 minute sessions per week produces a modest amount of weight loss of three to six pounds in one year. (Orzano AJ, Scott JC (2004). *JABFP*. 17(5) 359-369.)

The benefits of exercise cannot be measured in weight loss alone, as discussed in other sections of this book. Diet and exercise together provide greater weight loss than either one alone, as shown by studies of up to two years' duration. (Skender ML, Goodrick GK, Del Junco DJ, et al. (1996). *J Am Diet Assoc*. 96:342-346.)

Behavior therapy consists of behavior modification directed towards diet and exercise. This means counseling the patient regarding a healthy lifestyle, setting goals, self-monitoring towards these goals, and willpower. It's difficult to evaluate behavior therapy alone, since the goal is to get the patient on a healthy diet and exercising.

The final subject is drug therapy. The role of drug therapy in obesity is controversial, since most patients regain their lost weight once the drug is discontinued. The decision to initiate drug therapy requires careful evaluation of risks and benefits. Drugs can help a patient lose body fat when used with both diet and exercise. Candidates for drug therapy include those who are unable to diet and/or exercise; those with a BMI greater than 30 kg/m2; those with a BMI of 27 to 29.9 kg/m2 with comorbidities such as diabetes and coronary artery disease; those for whom gastrointestinal bypass surgery is being considered; and those on whom essential surgery cannot technically be performed due to the high risk caused by morbid obesity.

The Doctor's Dilemma—Officer Tom's Story

Tom is a 42-year-old police officer initially weighing 245 pounds and measuring six feet in height. His initial BMI of 33.2 placed him in the obese category. He had gained 50 pounds over the last three years, and his recent physical exam and blood tests revealed the onset of hypertension, hyperlipidemia and early type 2 diabetes. His police chief had recently required that all officers pass a fitness test designed to simulate a foot pursuit and aiding an injured officer. Tom did not pass the fitness test, and so his job was in jeopardy.

Tom's goal was to lose 50 pounds and pass the test. I referred him to a weight-loss clinic, where he was placed on approximately 1,000 calories per day—200 grams of protein and 50 grams of carbohydrate. Proteins were confined exclusively to beef, chicken, fish, lean pork and eggs. Carbohydrates were restricted to fruits and vegetables. Tom was instructed to take an appetite suppressant consisting of phentermine and topiramate. He was monitored at weekly clinic visits, and Tom kept a daily diary of his diet and activity.

Within six weeks' time, Tom had lost 30 pounds and his BMI had dropped to 29.2. He was no longer obese. His blood tests and blood pressure showed improvement, and he was able to pass the fitness test. Was this a good result? Would pills for hypertension, diabetes and statins be a better option? Tom was healthier and happier. The ultimate benefit depends upon what happens next. He had the essential requirements for success: a goal to lose 50 pounds; a daily diary to monitor success; the discipline necessary to follow the program; and weekly clinic visits where he was in the company of like-minded people. Can Tom continue this program in the future? Are long-term appetite suppressants his best option?

This is the "doctor's dilemma" of short-term success with fasting, appetite suppressants and frequent office visits. The ideal approach is patient knowledge, patient discipline, and a healthy patient lifestyle of healthy food choices and exercise. I would have recommended a slower approach, permitting muscle growth and simultaneous fat loss over a longer time period. If Tom had measured his percent body fat and muscle mass, he would have found that a significant loss of muscle mass had accompanied his 30 pound weight loss. Questions regarding best treatment remain unanswered, since Tom has achieved his goals and is content.

We do not live in an ideal world, and human behavior, as discussed earlier, is governed by both emotions (fast, impulsive thinking) and objectivity (slow, deliberate thinking). Your doctor can't monitor your behavior every day, nor can he take you to the grocery store or bring you to the gym. My guess is that Tom might increase his exercise and remain on a healthy diet, *or* he might regain all the weight he lost and return to the weight loss clinic to repeat the program.

Appetite Suppressants

Phentermine

There are seven main FDA-approved drug options used in the treatment of obesity. For a new drug to be approved by the FDA, it must be tested against a placebo and show weight loss equal to or greater than 5% weight loss at one year, or show that 35% of patients achieve 5% weight loss and must achieve twice the loss of the placebo patients.

Phentermine is a commonly used drug, owing to its efficacy and low price. This drug was approved by the FDA in 1959, and since it became generic, there has been little research done on this drug. Phentermine is an amphetamine-like drug that suppresses the appetite by acting on several brain nuclei in the hypothalamus. Outside the brain, phentermine causes fat cells to break down fat by releasing epinephrine and norepinephrine.

Diethylpropion

Diethylpropion is an amphetamine-like drug with minor sympathomimetic properties and fewer stimulant effects than phentermine. The FDA approved diethylpropion in 1959 for the treatment of obesity. A meta-analysis that assessed the use of diethylpropion for weight loss in obese individuals identified 13 studies published between 1965 and 1983. Obese patients treated lost an average of three kilograms of additional weight as compared to those on a placebo. (Haddock CK, et al. (2002). Int J Obes Relat Metab Disord. 26:262–273.)

Diethylpropion's approval was based on 69 patients randomized to diethylpropion 50 mg twice daily or placebo for six months. After this period, all participants received diethylpropion in an open-label extension for an additional six months. After the initial six months, the diethylpropion group lost an average of 9.8% of initial body weight vs. 3.2% in the placebo group. (Cercato C, et al. (2009). *Int J Obes (Lond).* 33:857–865.)

Common side-effects of diethylpropion include insomnia, dry mouth, dizziness, headache, mild increases in blood pressure, palpitations and rash.

Phenteramine and Toperamide

The combination of phentermine and toperamide (brand name "Qsymia") is a powerful appetite suppressant and has been FDA-approved since 2012. Phentermine has been discussed and is FDA-approved for short-term treatment of obesity, while topiramate is approved for non-weight-loss indications such as seizure disorders and migraine therapy. The amount of weight loss achieved with combination therapy is of greater magnitude than what could be achieved with either agent alone, and the combination may be taken for up to one year. (Shin JH, Gadde KM (2013). *Diabetes Metab Syndr Obes.* 6:131–

139. Published online 2013 Apr 8.)

Lorcaserin

Lorcaserin (Belviq) is a 5-HT2c serotonin receptor agonist that decreases appetite by acting directly on these receptors in the brain. It cannot be used with any drug that alters the metabolism of serotonin, such as selective serotonin reuptake inhibitors, tricyclic antidepressants, bupropion, triptans, St. John's Wort, tryptophan, or drugs that impair metabolism of serotonin (including monoamine oxidase inhibitors), dextromethorphan, lithium, tramadol, antipsychotics or other dopamine antagonists. Both lorcaserin and phentermine-topiramate have been approved for long-term weight loss, based on one-year trials showing that on top of recommendations to follow a calorie-restricted diet and increase exercise, patients randomized to either drug lost more weight than patients randomized to placebo (3%) as compared to lorcaserin (7%-8%) or phenteremine-toperamate (7%). (Woloshin S, Schwartz LM (April 2014). *JAMA Intern Med.* 174(4):615-619.)

These two drugs have been associated with side effects. Both drugs' labels include warnings regarding memory, attention, language problems and depression; lorcaserin's label also warns of valvular heart disease and euphoria; and the label for phentermine-topiramate warns of metabolic acidosis, increased heart rate, anxiety, insomnia and elevated creatinine levels.

Orlistat

Orlistat is a lipase inhibitor that prevents fat absorption in the gut. It is available without a prescription. Orlistat prevents the absorption of 30% of ingested fat. (Hauptman JB, Jeunet FS, Hartmann D. (1992). *Am J Clin Nutr.* 55(1):309S–313S.) Orlistat is dispensed as Xenical, 120 mg, three times daily. The side-effects are substantial and include stool incontinence, fecal urgency, flatus and fecal spotting. Orlistat is not the best treatment option, owing to its unpleasant side-effects.

Liraglutide

The fourth useful drug is liraglutide (Saxenda), an injectable glucagon-like peptide that increases insulin production and decreases appetite. Its side-effects include nausea and diarrhea. It is useful in patients with both diabetes and obesity. This seems contradictory, since one would expect that an increase in insulin would cause an increase in fat production. The mechanism of action is not completely understood, but likely depends on direct uptake of liraglutide by the arcuate nucleus in the hypothalamus. The centrally projecting neurons in the arcuate nucleus are important in the regulation of appetite and, when activated, they inhibit feeding. These neurons are activated by leptin and insulin.

Naltrexone and Bupropion

The combination of naltrexone and bupropion is called "Contrave." Naltrexone is an opioid antagonist that has been approved to treat opiod and alcohol dependency. It augments the action of bupropion. Bupropion is a dopamine and norepinephrine reuptake inhibitor approved for depression and smoking addiction. It activates nuclei in the hypothalamus (brain) that decrease appetite and food cravings. This combination does not have any cardiac contraindications, but does cause an increased rate of depression and suicide. One cannot drink alcohol or take opioid pain medications when taking Contrave.

Herbs

Herbal treatments, such as garcinia cambogia, have not been found to be useful in the treatment of obesity. (Heymsfield SB, Allison DB, Vasselli JR, Pietrobelli A, Greenfield D, Nunez C. (1998). *JAMA*. 280: 1596– 1600.)

In Summary

My criticism of my medical colleagues is very simple. Each FDA-approved use of a prescription drug for the treatment of obesity is preceded by the general statement, "when diet and exercise alone do not work" or "to be used with diet and exercise." This statement is never objectively controlled nor quantified: how much exercise was performed? What was the calorie and macronutrient content of the diet? Was there a daily diary? Is the data a subjective verbal report by patient?

My colleagues know that the benefits of prescription drug therapy occur only during such drug therapy, and that weaning patients off of these drugs then leads to weight gain in the absence of diet and exercise. (Yanovski SZ, Yanovski JA (2014). *JAMA* 311(1):74-86.) This is the benefit of short-term gain and the frustration of long-term loss.

What is missing is patient education. Patients must learn about diet and exercise so that they can be in control of and do something about their situation, and gain motivation for long-term success. Nobody wishes to change their comfortable lifestyle if they can achieve their goals by just taking a pill. Physicians don't have the ability to control the patient's environment, and are thus unable to objectively control what a patient eats and what exercises a patient performs.

The successful treatment of obesity requires a long-term lifestyle change, as well as cultural change—knowledge, diet and exercise. These do not come inside a bottle of pills.

CHAPTER 10
EVOLUTION, PROGRESS, CHANGE

You Were Born to Exercise

We are Homo sapiens, and our species evolved from archaic species in the Middle Awash of Ethiopia, per objective fossil evidence. According to Rebecca Cann, the region where people have lived the longest should have the greatest genetic diversity—and Africa has the greatest genetic diversity.

Based on mitochondrial DNA evidence, we are all related to a woman who lived in Africa 100,000 to 200,000 years ago. The Middle Awash region of Ethiopia may be the place where people have lived the longest. Fossil evidence in the area reveals the presence of hominids (erect bipedal primates) who predate modern humans and are likely our immediate ancestors. (White TD, et al. (2003). *Nature*. 423:742-747.)

Early hominids were not the dominant species but, rather, were hunted as prey. What changes were necessary for modern humans to become the dominant species as we are today? A reasonable theory based on fossil and anatomic evidence is that the adaptation to long-distance running improved food scavenging, thus increasing brain size and the subsequent dominance of Homo sapiens—the human species.

Early hominids could walk, but their skeletons suggest that they could not run well. The early species were adapted to tree dwelling, with long toes and an appositional first foot digit (thumb). Modern toes are short and straight, and are more energy-efficient for running. Modern human legs are longer relative to body mass, decreasing the energy expended while running. The modern human plantar arches and Achilles tendons provide sources of elastic, spring-like energy useful only when running.

Most animal species can run faster than can humans, but most cannot run *farther*. Most medium to large mammals pant to prevent over-heating while running. Modern humans sweat to prevent overheating, and this is done over a greater body surface area and is thus more efficient.

The theory of "persistence hunting" is that modern humans used endurance running to drive animals into hyperthermia and thus be more easily hunted. (Pickering TR, Bunn HT (2007). *J Human Evol.* 53(4):434-438.)

Thus, all modern humans have a body uniquely adapted, over thousands of years, to endurance exercise. What your body is unable to do is adapt to a sedentary, "modern" lifestyle; therefore, more people today are suffering from chronic metabolic diseases.

According to the National Institute on Aging, there has been a dramatic increase in average life expectancy during the 20th century. Most babies born in 1900 did not live past the age of 50. Life expectancy at birth in the U.S. (as of 2012) now exceeds 78 years.

The real question is, are we living *better* lives? The National Center for Biological Technology Information states, "The leading risk factors related to disability life years were dietary risks, tobacco smoking, high body mass index, high blood pressure, high fasting plasma glucose, physical inactivity, and alcohol use." In simple terms, metabolic disabilities in the U.S. comprise a larger share of life expectancy. We are not adapting well to our longer lives, and the problem is not simply aging, but rather personal lifestyle choices.

James Fries made this very clear in his classic 50 year study of 1,741 people at the University of Pennsylvania. (Vita AJ, et al. (1998). *New England J Med*. 338:1035-1041.) Cumulative lifetime disability was four times greater in those who smoked, were obese, and did not exercise than it was in those who did not smoke, were lean, and exercised.

According to Fries, despite the current reduction in smoking today, there is still an increase in obesity in the U.S. and the percentage of people who exercise has remained stable. Thus, we, as a nation, could be healthier if more of us exercised and ate an intelligent diet.

Not all scientists and physicians agree that diet and exercise alone will make us healthier. Questions regarding exactly how caloric restriction prolongs longevity remain unanswered.

We will never be able to do a controlled prospective long-term study of caloric restrictions in humans, because it would be considered unethical; we can study this subject in primates and lesser species only.

There has only been one such prospective controlled primate study completed, done at the University of Wisconsin from 1989 to 2009. This study clearly showed that calorie restriction increased longevity by 56.2%. (Colman RJ, et al. (2014). *Nature Communications*. 5:3557.) How to explain this is still being debated and studied.

There are negative effects of caloric restriction which depend on the degree of starvation. During World War II, a group of lean men restricted their calorie intake by 45% for six months, and ate mostly carbohydrates. (Keys A, et al. (1950). *The Biology of Human Starvation*, Vol. 2:1133.) This "starvation" resulted in many positive metabolic changes: decreased body fat; lower blood pressure; lower serum cholesterol; lower resting heart rate; and a lower daily caloric resting expenditure (REE). This caloric restriction also had negative effects: anemia, swollen lower extremities due to lower serum proteins; muscle weakness; lethargy; and depression. These negative effects were also caused by the lack of protein and fat in this unhealthy, predominantly carbohydrate (90%) diet. The question remains: "What caused the beneficial effects"?

We have already discussed reactive oxygen species (ROS), also called free radicals. In the presence of high blood glucose/sugar levels—such as when overeating—mitochondria in all cells become less efficient and must work harder. These stressed mitochondria produce more ROS. The increased ROS then cause more damage to our DNA, and kill more cells.

In the presence of calorie restriction and low blood glucose levels our mitochondria work less, are more efficient, and produce less ROS. Thus, there is less DNA damage, fewer cells are killed, and we live longer.

Today, there is great interest in finding drugs or supplements that will prolong life span and emulate in humans the same effects of calorie restriction but *without* the calorie restriction. Calorie restriction activates certain genes (SIR2 and PNC1). These genes are the targets of this new area of drug research. (de Magalhaes JP, et al. (2012). *Pharmacol Rev.* 64:88-101.)

To date, no drug nor supplement has been found that mimics the beneficial effects of calorie restriction. What does this mean to you? It means that you still need to exercise and diet intelligently in order to have a healthy lifestyle.

Modern Society and Hunter-Gatherers

Hunter-gatherers obtain their food by hunting wild animals and gathering wild plants. For most of human history, hunting and gathering were how we obtained our food. Farming and domestication of animals eventually replaced hunting and gathering in nearly all parts of the world. Today, just a small number of hunter-gatherers remains, and it is instructive to compare the health of modern society to that of modern hunter-gatherers.

Some hunger-gatherers can be found in the Americas, Africa and Asia. If we compare a simple health marker—such as blood pressure—it appears that modern hunter-gatherers are healthier than is our modern industrialized population.

Progress is the Root of All Evil—How Our Modern Lifestyle Changed Our Health

In 1956, my mother took me to see the play "Li'l Abner." This musical, based on the comic strip *Li'l Abner*, contains a song called "Progress is the Root of All Evil." I didn't understand this refrain when I was 12 years old, and now—many years later—I understand what Johnny Mercer was saying.

With regard to our bodies and health, modern society has given us many new problems. Thousands of years ago, when hunter-gatherers became sedentary farmers, they were able to grow more food and domesticate farm animals. This abundance of calories allowed women to increase their birth rate. The average birth rate of sedentary farmers is estimated to be double that of hunter-gatherers. (Appel B, et al. (2011). *Science*. 560-561.) Farm children became farmers, as well, and populations grew, as did the abundance of food, leading to cities, free time, art and culture.

Sedentary farmers tend to grow mostly carbohydrates (corn in some cultures), leading to a diet higher in carbohydrates than in the diets of hunter-gatherers. The Industrial Revolution of 1760 to 1840 essentially replaced the use of human muscle with machines. Our society changed, our diet changed to include more carbohydrates, and we used less and needed less muscle. Most people will continue to drive their cars to work and continue to use elevators; few will choose to walk. However, our metabolism remains unchanged, and this is the problem.

Modern society has more metabolic health problems than did our ancient ancestors, as we demonstrated above—hypertension, diabetes, heart disease and stroke—all owing to our unhealthy modern lifestyle. We still have basically the same type of body as did our ancient hunter-gatherer ancestors, but we live in a culture with dangerous food options and fewer requirements for muscular strength.

The best we can do is to understand how our body works, and give our body the lifestyle it needs in order to remain healthy in these dangerous modern times.

Blood Pressure

One important measure of your overall health is your blood pressure (BP), and we can use this measure to compare relative health between our modern society and contemporary hunter-gatherers.

The heart pumps blood into the arteries (blood vessels that convey blood to all parts of the body). When the heart muscle (left ventricle) contracts, the pressure created to push blood out into the arteries is the "systolic" or first number of a blood pressure reading (measured in millimeters of mercury). Normal systolic blood pressure is below 120.

When your heart muscle relaxes between beats, the pressure maintained in your arteries is the "diastolic" blood pressure. A normal diastolic blood pressure is below 80.

Blood pressure is reported using both the systolic and diastolic numbers: "120/80." An elevated blood pressure, such as 140/95, is called hypertension. In general, the lower your blood pressure, the longer you will live.

Men and women with hypertension have a shorter life expectancy and a higher risk of coronary artery disease, myocardial infarction and stroke. (Franco OH, et al. (2005). *Hypertension.* 46(2):280-286.)

In one study, normotensive men and women survives 7.2 years longer without cardiovascular disease compared to hypertensive men and women, and spent 2.1 fewer years of life with cardiovascular disease. Compared to hypertensives, total life expectancy was longer for both normotensive men and women. Increased blood pressure in adulthood is associated with reduction in life expectancy.

Blood pressure readings of modern hunter-gatherers are well below the modern industrialized average of <120/<80: Bushmen at 108/63;Yanomamo at 104/65; Xingu at 107/68; and Kitava at 113/71. (Carrera-Bastos P et al. (2011). *Research Reports in Clinical Cardiology.* 211(2):15-35.) In addition, blood pressure does not increase with age as it does in North Americans.

Other health marker improvements in the hunter-gatherers include increased insulin sensitivity, lower plasma insulin levels, lower leptin levels, lower BMI, smaller waist size, and lower skinfold measurements. It appears that our modern lifestyle has made our bodies less healthy.

Why We Continue to Eat "Bad" Food

As a society, we continue to eat "bad" food because we aren't critical in our food choices, and we don't use the knowledge that's outlined in this book.

Here are three additional reasons we make bad food choices:

The first is that the obesity epidemic in this country has been aided by the low cost of high glucose-containing carbohydrates. These foods (soy beans and corn) are inexpensive because their production and storage is subsidized by the U.S. government in the Farm Bill. For the past 50 years, U.S. farm policy has been directed towards driving down the price of farmed storable carbohydrates (again, corn and soybeans).

At the same time, the cost of growing fruits and vegetables has increased, as has their retail price. Low costs incentivizes the food industry to use more of these unhealthy commodities. High-fructose corn syrup is now commonly added to many foods (*processed* foods).

In summary, the food industry has a huge financial incentive to make food with high-glycemic carbohydrates.

The second reason we eat "bad" food is due to marketing. "Marketing" is defined as "whatever it takes to make you buy a specific product."

One of the most useful marketing techniques is to aim marketing messages at children, who then nag their parents to buy this or that product; then, the child may continue to buy that product well into adulthood.

The food industry spends over $1.6 billion dollars marketing food to children. (HBO documentary series *The Weight of the Nation*, May 2012.) Most of these products are processed foods which are high in calories and sugar, and often lead to obesity.

Every month, approximately 90% of American children between the ages of three to nine years visit a McDonalds. (*Fast Food Nation*, Schlosser E, Mariner Books, Houghton Mifflin Harcourt, 2012.) Is it a coincidence that McDonalds operates over 8,000 restaurant-playgrounds? (Schlosser E (1/17/2001) *Fast Food Nation: The Dark Side of the All-American Meal*, p. 35, Houghton Mifflin Harcourt, Kindle edition.)

Fast-food chains profit when children drink soda, because soda has the highest profit margin. Today, McDonald's sells more Coca-Cola® than anyone else in the world. A medium Coke that sells for $1.29 contains roughly 9 cents' worth of syrup. (Schlosser E (1/17/2001). *Fast Food Nation: The Dark Side of the All-American Meal*, p. 42, Houghton Mifflin Harcourt, Kindle edition.)

The third reason we continue to eat poorly is the belief that "labels do not lie." Marketing companies have created labels using a selection of words that make us believe we are eating healthy food when, in fact, we are *not*.

"Whole grain" refers to a cereal product containing the germ, endosperm and bran, and thus *not* refined or man-made. Yet, the stamp "whole grain" from the Whole Grains Council means the product must contain only 8 grams of whole grain per 30 grams of product, and thus is mostly *not* comprised of whole grains. The label stating "Made With Whole Grain" actually may mean that only a tiny amount of whole grain is present.

The label "Heart Healthy," sold by the American Heart Association for use on foods, refers to the fat and salt content of a product but *not* the sugar content of the product; thus, one real cause of heart disease is not even accounted for.

The term "all natural" really should be labeled "stay away!" The USDA does not define foods labeled "all natural" as any different than those labeled "natural." Foods with this labeling are usually not any different than "natural" foods, and may not be regulated, as they are not defined by the USDA. Foods labeled "natural," according to the USDA definition, do not contain artificial ingredients or preservatives, and the ingredients are only minimally processed. However, they may contain antibiotics, growth hormones, and other similar chemicals. People often confuse "natural" with "organic"; they are not the same, nor are they on a par with each other.

CHAPTER 11

SUMMARY: HOW TO IMPROVE YOUR HEALTH

IN 12 STEPS

1. In your web browser, visit Mayo Clinic's calorie calculator (you can find it at www.mayoclinic.org/healthy-lifestyle/nutrition-and-healthy-eating/in-depth/calorie-calculator/itt-20084939).

2. Calculate how many calories you need every day, and then subtract 500 calories. Use the resulting number as an approximation of your daily caloric limit in order to target one pound of weight loss per week—no more than one pound per week. Any small loss is good.

3. Calculate your protein needs based on your weight in pounds. Start your diet with 1 gram of protein per pound of body weight; this will provide your daily protein and fat.

4. Calculate the calorie content of your protein meals by weighing your food on a food scale or using package labels.

5. Daily diet calories minus protein and fat calories equals

carbohydrate calories. This resulting number is the number of calories you should obtain from carbohydrates.

6.   Select healthy foods, as described in this book. Eat all the vegetables and salads that you can—the more fiber the better; these calories do not count.

7.   Weigh yourself every day, and keep a written or electronic journal. Measure your waist size once a month.

8.   Do 30 to 40 minutes of vigorous cardiovascular exercise three to five times per week—treadmill, elliptical, bike, running, jogging, swimming.

9.   Resistance-train each muscle group once a week—pushing on Monday, legs on Wednesday, pulling on Friday, with a rest day in between. Your muscles grow during these rest periods.

10. Sleep well, and allow your body to recover. Rest, without engaging in any exercise, one or two days per week; don't exercise every single day.

11. Expect your body to change slowly. You must change your diet and exercise program in order to continue to improve slowly—it's a race that's won by the turtle.

12. Say "show me the data!" to anyone giving you health advice.

THE AUTHORS

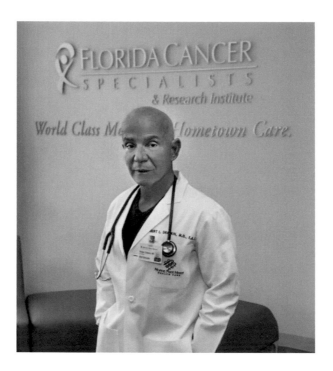

Robert Drapkin, MD, FACP

Robert Drapkin, MD, FACP

I am the son of a poor boy born in the town of Polotsk, Belarus, around 1900. My dad lifted himself out of poverty with sheer determination and hard work so that he could attend medical school at the University of Bern, Switzerland. He became a general practitioner of medicine (MD) in Albany, New York, and raised me, his only son. I was predestined to go to medical school; it was expected, and there were no other options in my life in Albany.

I look back with appreciation of my dad's guidance. I accepted early admission at Wayne State Medical School in Detroit, Michigan. I wanted to get away from New York State, where my dad had some influence.

In 1967, Wayne State was the only medical school in Detroit, and the clinical experience was intense. Every howling ambulance brought me a new problem to solve.

I did my internship and residency at the University of Illinois in Chicago—another trauma hospital with an active emergency room. I lived and breathed medicine; it was my entire life, and I loved it.

I became the Chief Resident and Instructor in Medicine my last year in Chicago, and then accepted a fellowship in Medical Oncology at Memorial Sloan Kettering in New York City. I enjoyed Oncology, as it was complicated and interesting internal medicine.

My next academic role was as a full-time attending and assistant professor at Roswell Park Memorial Institute in Buffalo, New York—a New York State-managed oncology center. I always felt more comfortable at the bedside than in the laboratory, and I subsequently moved to the west coast of Florida in 1979, where the incidence of cancer was high and the oncology resources were few.

In summary, I've been an MD since 1971. I've been taking care of sick folks in an academic setting and in private practice for over 45 years. I learned almost everything I know from my patients.

Dr. Drapkin's Current Gym Training Schedule

I weigh 140 pounds. I train one hour per day, four days per week, in a commercial gym. I recommend not building a home gym, because part of your motivation comes from the other people in the gym—you watching other people exercise, and other people watching you exercise. There's always much to learn from others, and new data is constantly forthcoming.

Two hours before training, I eat a 500-calorie breakfast containing 38 grams of protein, 40 grams of carbohydrate and approximately 20 grams of fat.

Before lifting any weights, I do myofascial release with a foam roller on the target muscles for that day, as well as dynamic active and passive stretching with my trainer. I perform core-strengthening exercises.

I drink copious amounts of water throughout the hour of exercise.

Monday: I target the pushing muscles of the chest, shoulders and triceps, followed by the abdominal muscles and ending with core exercises. I take branch chain amino acids and L citrulline immediately following the exercise, and my second meal of the day is 30 minutes later.

1. Chest press with a slight 30 degree incline bench with barbells or dumbbells—three sets.

2. Chest press, as above, with a 45 degree incline or machine press—three sets (may do five second negatives).

3. Military press—a 90 degree incline, as above, or machine—three sets (may do five second negatives).

4. Triceps rope pull-downs and skull crushers with barbell—three sets.

5. Abdominal crunches with a 25 lb dumbbell resting on Bosu. All sets are done to muscle failure. If it's possible to do 12 repetitions, the weight is increased with a target of six repetitions. For fewer than six repetitions, the weight is decreased. We aim for a one or two-minute rest between sets.

Wednesday is leg day:

1. Smith machine squats—four sets.

2. Inclined leg press—three sets followed by a drop set.

3. Leg extensions by machine.

4. Leg curls by machine.

5. Posterior chain back extensions.

Friday is back, trapezius and biceps day:

1. Pull-ups—three sets.

2. Horizontal cable row—three sets.

3. High cable row—three sets.

4. Mid-back inverted rows or dumbbell mid-back rows—three sets.

5. Trapezius Smith machine pull-ups—three sets.

6. Barbell biceps curls—four sets.

7. Abdominal crunches.

8. Core—planks on stability ball or foam roller and ball rollouts.

Saturday is posterior chain leg and arms day:

1. Deadlifts.

2. Single-leg inclined leg press.

3. Triceps rope pull-downs alternating with seated dumbbell biceps curls.

4. Abdominal hanging leg pull-ups and Bosu crunches.

5. Core—planks on stability ball or foam roller and ball rollouts.

I do cardio two to three days per week—30 minutes of HIIT on my bicycle or elliptical machine—on the days that I don't lift weights.

That's all, folks!

—Robert Louis Drapkin, MD, FACP

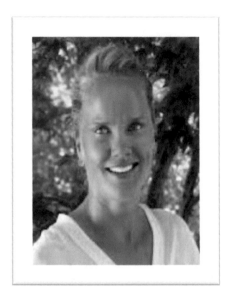

Ashleigh Gass, MS, CSCS, CCN, CNS, CISSN

Ashleigh Gass, MS, CSCS, CCN, CNS, CISSN

Ashleigh Gass, MS, CSCS, CCN, CNS, CISSN's extensive credentials include a master's degree in Human/Clinical Nutrition through the University of Bridgeport; Certified Sports Nutritionist through the International Society of Sports Nutrition (CISSN); Certified Clinical Nutritionist (CCN); and Certified Nutrition Specialist (CNS). She is also a Certified Strength and Conditioning Specialist (CSCS) and Medical Exercise Specialist (MES), as well as a Certified Level One CrossFit Coach. She is currently working within the GymnasticBodies™ system as an athlete and coach.

Ashleigh graduated from the University of Victoria, British Columbia, in 2003. She earned her BS studying kinesiology, exercise physiology and psychology. Ashleigh is also a graduate of the National Coaching Institute, having completed extensive sports science modules in the long-term physical preparation of the elite athlete.

Ashleigh has worked with weekend warriors, college athletes and high-level competitors for over 10 years. Her work has included positions as the exercise therapist and physical preparation coach for

Synergy Health Management in her native British Columbia. She also provided years of strength and conditioning coaching for the Camosun College Chargers men's and women's basketball teams and men's volleyball team; the 2004 Men's U23 national rugby team; and the 2004 World Junior Taekwondo Championships in Korea.

Ashleigh brings her wealth of education and experience to Brilliant Fitness and Nutrition (BFN), formerly Brilliant Athlete, and uses it to create a culture that is focused on success, measurable results, hard work, fun, and ownership of outcomes. She brings cutting-edge training and nutrition solutions to her clients to help them achieve their wellness and performance goals. She's well-known in the Tampa Bay area for her results-based coaching style.

Ashleigh is an accomplished natural body building and figure show competitor. She won the overall title at the 2010 Hurricane Bay Championship, and consistently places in the top three in national qualifying shows in Florida. Her pursuit of excellence in the figure world is a convenient spin-off of her training and healthy lifestyle.

Her training methods and competitive wins have been profiled in several respected health and fitness publications. Ashleigh is also a published writer, providing articles about training and nutrition to numerous local publications. She has presented at national conferences, including the International Society of Sports Nutrition Conference (ISSN) in June, 2010. Ashleigh launched Brilliant Fitness and Nutrition (BFN), formerly Brilliant Athlete in 2008, in Los Angeles, and then brought her company and expertise to the Tampa/Clearwater area. Her resume is available upon request.

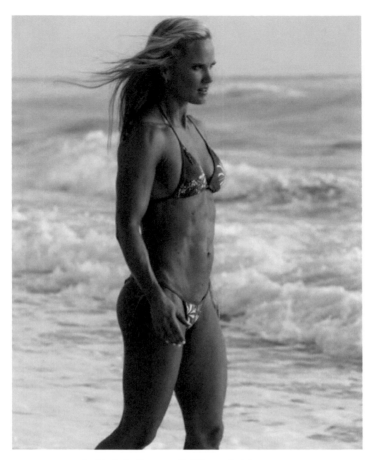

Ashleigh Gass—Brilliant Athlete

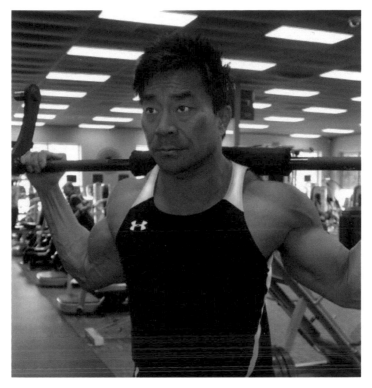

Donny H. Kim, Master Trainer, PES, CPT-NASM.

Donny H. Kim, Master Trainer, PES, CPT-NASM

Donny H. Kim, Master Trainer, PES, CPT-NASM, was born in 1966 in Seoul, Korea. When his father's commercial trucking business came to a crashing halt in 1976, his family immigrated to the U.S., seeking a better life. Donny was 10 years old at the time; he literally learned the alphabet and how to write his name in English just days before moving.

The language and cultural barriers were tough on the entire family, and especially for Donny's father. They first settled in Edgar, Nebraska, from 1976 until 1978. It was a tiny town located in south-central Nebraska, mostly comprised of hard-working German descendants. There were no other Korean families within a 50 mile radius. Looking back, Donny finds that this really helped them to become integrated into their new world. He still remembers his father's words: "Be a great representation of yourself, your family and your nationality." He expressed that they needed to not just be better, but to be way better, in their new world. Donny's father also encouraged the family to excel in everything they did.

In 1978, the family moved to Michigan City, Indiana, where Donny's father had a distant relative. All through school, Donny thrived in academics and sports, as well as leadership positions. He graduated with numerous high honors and highest varsity sport points, and served as the senior high school class president. He had ROTC and wrestling scholarships available, but decided to take the academic scholarship at Indiana University.

Donny did his undergraduate studies and attended law school at I.U. Bloomington. Starting in 1985, he oversaw the Student Athletic Center, and he entered his first bodybuilding competition, which he loved. Soon thereafter, he realized that a law career was his father's goal for him, and he found his passion in fitness and coaching. So, after law school, he did everything he could find in the fitness business—presale, front desk, training, sales, and even general manager.

In late 1995, he relocated to Tampa Bay. Between 1995 and 2012, he became the top personal trainer and training manager for both Gold's Gym and Lifestyle Family Fitness. During this time, he won numerous bodybuilding titles, including Mr. Tampa Bay, Mr. Florida Natural and World Superbody Runner-Up—Lightweight; he also earned the status of Professional Natural Bodybuilder.

Donny has modeled and acted and, more importantly, served Tampa Bay as a fitness and nutrition expert. In 2012, he started Tampa Bay Fitness, and continues to serve as its president.

Donny has an incredible home life with his beautiful wife, Angela, and his amazing son, Michael, who share his success, joy and happiness. Put simply, he loves what he does. He has happy clients, is respected by his peers, and makes his living by helping others.

As of the time of this writing, Donny has been in the fitness industry for 30 years—and he's still happily exhausted every day. He hopes to continue to reach more and more people with his knowledge and passion.

Donny can be reached at donnykimfit@gmail.com or (727) 410-9210.